LIBERTY GARDENS
—GUIDEBOOK—

LIBERTY GARDENS
—GUIDEBOOK—

**A Beginner's Guide to Freedom and
Flourishing Through Growing Healthy Food**

RANDAL CLARK

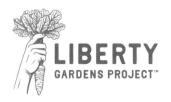

LIBERTY
GARDENS PROJECT™

For all the Liberty Gardeners yet to come. May your garden—and your life—flourish.

Cover and illustrations: Weylon Smith
Editorial: Rachel Miller

Publisher's Cataloging-in-Publication Data

Names: Clark, Randal, author.
Title: Liberty gardens guidebook : a beginner's guide to freedom and flourishing through growing healthy food / Randal Clark.
Description: Franklin, TN: Liberty Gardens Project, 2024.
Identifiers: LCCN: 2024924611 | ISBN: 978-1-966368-01-4 (paperback) 9781966368007 (e-book)
Subjects: LCSH Vegetable gardening. | Kitchen gardens. | BISAC GARDENING / Garden Design | GARDENING / Techniques | GARDENING / Container | GARDENING / Vegetables
Classification: LCC SB453 .C53 2024 | DDC 635--dc23

CONTENTS

Become a Liberty Gardener
in Five Simple Steps

Additional Resources

WELCOME! LET'S DIG IN.

Hello, gardener!

"Hold up—I'm not a gardener!" you might be thinking. And technically, you might be right. But after working your way through this guide, we hope you change your mind (and have some veggies to show for it).

Here at Liberty Gardens Project, we believe in your innate human capacity to grow. Gardening is the oldest profession, and for most of history, it wasn't unusual to have a garden—it was unusual not to!

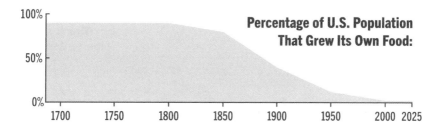

Our goal is to help you—and hundreds of thousands of other beginners like you—get out there and grow something.

We invite you to roll up your sleeves, get your hands dirty, and eagerly await the day when you eat something that came from your backyard. Not only will it be delicious, but it'll be served with a side of satisfaction—as you'll know how hard you worked to enjoy it.

Here's to the flourishing life!

Cheers,
Liberty Gardens Project

Grow something. Grow anything. Gardens everywhere.

WHAT IS A LIBERTY GARDEN?

At its core, a Liberty Garden gives you freedom. It gives you the power to cultivate the type of produce you want to eat and the quality of produce you deserve.

When you grow a Liberty Garden, you're not just starting a new hobby or riding the wave of an internet homesteading trend. You're joining a movement. You're plugging into a network of people who care deeply about their community, who crave nutritious food, who are tired of paying outrageous prices for mediocre (or worse—unhealthy) produce, and who have a sense of pride and confidence that comes from cultivating land and seeing results.

By starting a Liberty Garden, you're saying yes to a flourishing life.

A Liberty Garden isn't just for people who have an abundance of land. If you live in an apartment and can only grow a potted tomato plant on your patio, cheers to your Liberty Garden!

When we say "Grow something. Grow anything. Gardens everywhere," we mean it. In general, it's best to start small and scale anyway. Our simple model will help you learn as you go and expand your garden at the right time.

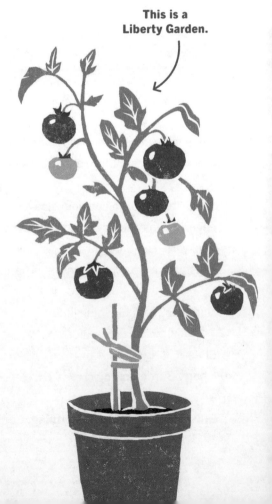

This is a Liberty Garden.

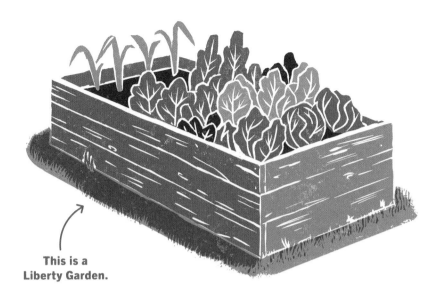

This is a
Liberty Garden.

That being said, if you have enough sunny space, **we recommend starting your Liberty Garden with one 4' x 8' raised bed**. This will provide you with a substantial amount of food to supplement your needs and reduce your grocery bill. You're also welcome to skip the bed and plant your garden directly in the ground—the bed just offers some conveniences when preparing your soil.

A garden is a great place for experimentation. Failure is part of the process, especially when you refuse to use toxic pesticides. Bugs, blights, and bad weather are inevitable. Go ahead and expect at least some failure—it means you're doing it right! After all, freedom is a bit messy, and it's fun to make a mess sometimes.

This is a
Liberty Garden.

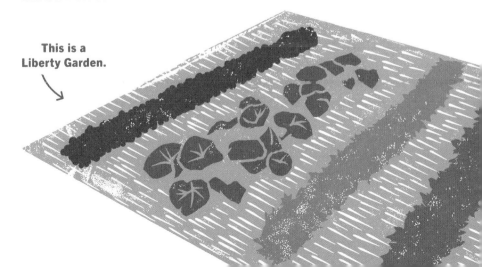

Why Build a 4' x 8' Raised Bed?

The Liberty Gardens 4' x 8' is intentionally designed with you in mind:

▸ **The shopping list is simple.** We've made it easy to shop for lumber at your local home improvement store—see the full shopping list on page 29.

▸ **No digging required.** A raised bed saves you the backbreaking work of tilling soil. All you've got to do is fill the bed with soil and compost.

▸ **Everything's within reach.** You'll never have to reach more than two feet in any direction to tend to your vegetables.

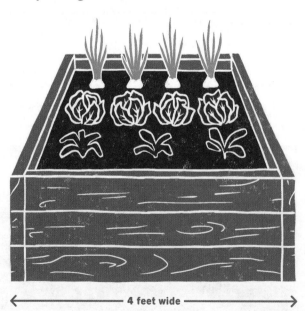

⟵————— 4 feet wide —————⟶

WHY GROW A LIBERTY GARDEN?

Allow us a 30-second sociology lesson. In governments ruled by monarchs, there's a term called *abdicating*, which is when a member of the family renounces his or her call to rule. Abdicating is opting out of your responsibility and giving your power to someone else.

With the rise of globalization and the mind-blowing advances in technology over the past couple of centuries, most of us have abdicated basic skills to institutions who do things we don't want to do ourselves. For example, why would you learn how to sew and make your own clothes when you can purchase a new outfit with a few clicks of a button? We've outsourced our responsibilities to hyperfocus on other, more "important" pursuits, like financial success or leisure time. But as it turns out, these pursuits aren't bringing us the flourishing life we thought they would.

We have surrendered our responsibility to nourish our own bodies. A Liberty Garden helps you take back your power.

Abdicating our responsibility to grow our own food has brought major unintended consequences. We've become dependent on institutions that don't have our best interests at heart. Food, water, energy, transportation, shelter, health care—we rely on the powers-that-be to take care of all our basic survival needs. And the more autonomy we yield, the more powerful they become.

The Food Challenges Before Us

When it comes to the food industry, the results speak for themselves. Our abdication has hurt our stomachs, our farmers, and the land we're called to cultivate. Take a look at some of the issues we're facing:

- ▸ **Food Scarcity and Insecurity:** In 2023, 13.5% of American households experienced food insecurity—meaning 18 million people struggled to meet their basic nutritional needs.[1] Households that can't find or afford healthy food suffer physical, emotional, educational, and financial consequences.

- ▸ **"Big Food" Monopolies:** Ten companies in the United States control 90% of the produce supply, and five companies control 90% of the meat supply. Consolidations can make supply unpredictable and can lead to fewer options for you and your family to choose from.

- ▸ **Poor Food Quality:** People in America are overfed and undernourished. The ultra-processed food we consume isn't just low in nutrition—in many cases, it's actually harming us. Plus, our industrial farming practices deplete the soil of its nutrients, causing diminishing returns in each new crop.

- ▸ **Fragile Supply Chains:** It's been a wild time for supply chains. World events of the past few years are a sobering reminder that food doesn't just magically appear on the grocery store shelves. Our complex global supply chains are all too easily shut down.

---

[1] "Food Security and Nutrition Assistance," U.S. Department of Agriculture, Economic Research Service, accessed November 17, 2024, https://www.ers.usda.gov/data-products/ag-and-food-statistics-charting-the-essentials/food-security-and-nutrition-assistance/.

- **Inflation and Price Uncertainty:** Over the past four years, grocery prices have skyrocketed by 25%.[2] And over a third of Americans say they're struggling to provide food for their households.[3] Gardening will help you cut back on your grocery bill.

- **Our National Health Crisis:** The most tragic proof of all exists in our own bodies. The evidence is overwhelming: Americans are getting sicker every year. Four in 10 U.S. adults are obese—not just overweight.[4] And nearly 4 in 10 Americans have a chronic disease, such as hypertension, diabetes, cancer, or heart disease.[5] Big Food and Big Pharma make more money off people who are addicted to bad food—keeping them stuck in a cycle of "health care" that focuses on relieving symptoms rather than getting to the root of the problem.

Most of us grew up taking food for granted. But these increasingly complicated factors have made us aware: What got us here won't get us to a flourishing life. We have surrendered our responsibility to nourish our own bodies. A Liberty Garden is a quiet rebellion in a culture of abdication, allowing you to take back your power.

[2] "Food Prices and Spending," U.S. Department of Agriculture, Economic Research Service, accessed November 17, 2024, https://www.ers.usda.gov/data-products/ag-and-food-statistics-charting-the-essentials/food-prices-and-spending/.

[3] "The State of Personal Finance: 2024," Ramsey Solutions, accessed November 17, 2024, https://www.ramseysolutions.com/budgeting/state-of-personal-finance.

[4] Samuel D. Emmerich, DVM., Cheryl D. Fryar, MSPH., Bryan Stierman, MD, MPH, and Cynthia L. Ogden, PhD, MRP, "Obesity and Severe Obesity Prevalence in Adults: United States, August 2021–August 2023" NCHS Data Brief, no. 508 (September 2024), https://www.cdc.gov/nchs/data/databriefs/db508.pdf.

[5] Gabriel A. Benavidez, PhD, Whitney E. Zahnd, PhD, Peiyin Hung, PhD, and Jan M. Eberth, PhD, "Chronic Disease Prevalence in the US: Sociodemographic and Geographic Variations by Zip Code Tabulation Area," Preventing Chronic Disease, no. 21 (February 2024), https://doi.org/10.5888/pcd21.230267.

We Did It Before, and We'll Do It Again

Liberty Gardens have roots in another type of garden: the Victory Garden.

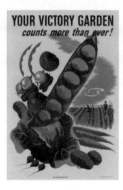

During World War II, the Department of Agriculture encouraged U.S. citizens to grow their own fruits and vegetables to ease food shortages and support troops overseas. These homegrown gardens fostered unity among those holding down the fort while loved ones served. The original Victory Garden guide proclaimed: "You may not be able to carry a gun or drive a tank, but you can grow food for victory!"

The results were astounding: **Over four years (1941–1945), Americans planted 20 million gardens, which provided 40% of the vegetables in the U.S.**[6]

Nearly a century later, we're facing a new and unique set of food challenges. Any effort to create something healthy will make a difference. By working together, we can change industries—and it's easier than you think. Liberty Gardens Project aims to make gardening simple and get you growing right away.

---

[6] "Time for Victory Gardens Again?" U.S. Department of Agriculture, Tellus, accessed November 17, 2024, https://tellus.ars.usda.gov/stories/articles/time-victory-gardens-again.

WHY WE GARDEN

Every gardener is unique. We all approach gardening with different motivations, hopes, and goals. We asked a few friends in our Liberty Garden community why they choose to garden, and here's what we found:

"I love knowing I can live off my land."

"It feels good to know I can provide for myself and my family—at least in part—without relying on anyone else. It's sustainable, too. I'm going to get better at it every season. The world feels kind of unpredictable these days, and I love the security that comes from knowing I can grow my own food."

— **Mike C.**

"I'm a foodie at heart."

"I mean . . . have you ever tasted food fresh from the soil? Like, a carrot that you pulled out of the ground, washed up, and enjoyed right then? Once you taste homegrown food, you'll be ruined for the grocery store stuff. Those fruits and veggies sit on the shelves for weeks—some literally for months—before you eat them. I guess I'm a snob and I just like eating the best food possible."

— **Blanca N.**

"Health matters to me."

"Gardening empowers me to know exactly what I'm putting in my body. No toxins, no preservatives, no microplastics or whatever other terrible things they're finding in foods these days. We can't afford to buy organic produce all the time, so I got fed up with it and decided to grow it myself!"

— **Ellie V.**

"It's a great hobby!"

"I got sick of being super boring and having no hobbies. So I took up gardening. Once, I watched this documentary about the blue zones—places in the world where people easily live to 100 years old. And gardening is a very common hobby in these parts of the world. So, I think I'm on the right track! Plus, gardening is how I trick myself to exercise."

— **Saundra M.**

"I love sharing what I've grown with people!"

"In my opinion, veggies taste best when shared. Keeping a garden has connected me to my community in very practical ways—I've struck up friendships with neighbors just from being outside more. I love harvesting food from my garden and dropping a bag on a friend's porch, or serving it to my family for dinner that night."

— **Alex C.**

"It's a great way to get my grandkids off their screens and connected to nature."

"Kids have so few opportunities to enjoy nature these days. I love getting my grandkids outside, off their screens, in the garden with their hands in the dirt. They ask so many questions—and I don't know the answer to even half of them! But I see how proud they feel when the seeds sprout. I see how excited they get when they harvest food (sometimes too early!). Nature has always been important to me, and I want to pass that connection along to my grandkids."

— **Beth P.**

The benefits of gardening are overwhelming. Plus, while it takes some effort, gardening isn't complicated. The Liberty Garden model is convenient, simple, and straightforward. We provide you with all the information, resources, and tools you need in a proven, step-by-step process—making it easy for you to plant, grow, and enjoy food from your own backyard.

What's Your *Why*?

✎ **Why are you excited to grow your own food? Write your thoughts below.**

....

....

Become a Liberty Gardener in Five Simple Steps:

1 **PLAN**

2 **PREPARE**

3 **PLANT**

4 **PRODUCE**

5 **PARTAKE**

Let's get growing.

PLAN

No harvest happens by accident. A thriving Liberty Garden begins with a purposeful plan.

We're sure your mind is full of questions, and we get it! This might feel like a lot to take in. Don't worry—we'll guide you through the process and keep it as simple as possible.

To start planning your Liberty Garden, read through the questions and answers below, and jot down your ideas in the spaces provided.

How much time will gardening take?

Early on, you'll need to dedicate a few afternoons or weekends to prepare your garden: shopping, assembling, laying the soil and compost, and planting. But after some focused, hard work, you can maintain a Liberty Garden in five minutes a day—or less!

If you're unsure how much time you can dedicate, start with just one 4' x 8' bed instead of multiple. You can always scale later.

✎ **Get out your calendar. In the space below, write down a few time blocks or full days in late winter that you could dedicate to preparing your garden.**

....

....

....

🖉 Envision what your five-minute daily gardening routine will look like once you're in the swing of things. Could you check it first thing in the morning or right after work? Write your ideas below:

....

....

....

How much will it cost me to start a Liberty Garden?

Similar to your time commitment, a Liberty Garden requires an initial investment of money when you begin. A ballpark number to budget is a couple hundred dollars for one 4' x 8' bed (depending on what supplies you already have).

But after the initial purchases—plus a couple of ongoing costs like compost and seeds—gardening is free. And few activities produce such a great return on your investment. The profit margins you'll get on your homegrown veggies are remarkable, especially for their quality and nutritional value. And the tools you buy up front can be used for years to come.

🖉 Is there room in your budget to buy the supplies you'll need for your garden? If not, what changes could you make?

....

....

....

✐ One way to save money and build community is to borrow from friends. Is there anyone you know who already gardens and could lend you some supplies?

....

....

....

....

What will I grow?

At Liberty Gardens Project, we believe in growing only what you find delicious. It does no good to labor over vegetables you and your family don't want to eat! We've provided sample plans for you to follow to grow the best foods for your region, but you should always customize them to your preferences.

✐ What are your favorite types of produce?

☐ Carrots   ☐ Broccoli

☐ Melons   ☐ Corn

☐ Garlic   ☐ Potatoes

☐ Lettuce   ☐ Basil

☐ Summer squash   ☐ Onions

☐ Radishes   ☐ Beans

☐ Cucumbers   ☐ Spinach

☐ Beets   ☐ Peppers

☐ Arugula   ☐ Kale

✏ Picture yourself seated around a table with friends or family eating a meal prepared with fresh vegetables from your garden. What does that experience look, feel, smell, and taste like? What foods would you like to serve them?

....

....

....

....

....

What supplies do I need?

✏ Explore your garage, shed, or utility closets. What gardening supplies (see pages 28–30) do you already have? Make note of what you'll need to purchase.

....

....

....

....

....

....

Where should I plant my garden?

First, your garden should get lots of sunshine—ideally, a full eight hours. Plant your rows north to south so the vegetables can receive even sun exposure throughout the day.

And second, your garden should be convenient for you to visit every day and water when needed. If at all possible, plant close to a hose spigot so you don't have to lug a watering can back and forth.

✏ **Head outside to your yard (and bring this book with you!). Scout out a few potential locations for your garden and write or draw them below.**

No Backyard! No Problem!

If you're living in an apartment or townhome, or if you're renting with restrictions on what you can do in your yard, here are a few creative solutions for growing a Liberty Garden:

▸ **Grow something—anything—in a single pot on your porch.** Pick one vegetable and just give it a go!

▸ **Use windowsill planter boxes.** If your space allows, try growing something right outside your window. You can find tons of windowsill boxes online or at your local gardening center.

▸ **Try the roof.** If you're in an apartment building, you might have access to roof space, which can be a great place to build your raised bed (if your management allows!).

▸ **Join a community garden.** Look for a community garden in your area. Make sure it's close enough to visit every day—or nearly every day.

▸ **Borrow some dirt.** If you've got a friend with some land, why not invite them to join your adventure? You can barter for the space by promising them a share of your harvest.

Who will help me?

Gardening isn't just about delicious food—it's about building a flourishing life. And friendships are key for flourishing. Gardening is a great way to strengthen existing friendships or make new ones. Whether it's a neighbor, a friend, your spouse, or your kids, consider inviting others to be a part of this journey.

✎ **Who would you like to invite to join you as you grow your Liberty Garden?**

....

....

....

....

....

Find Your Growing Zone and Garden Plan

Where you live has a huge impact on what you grow and how you grow it. The United States has a variety of growing zones—geographical areas with distinct temperatures, elevations, rainfall, and frost dates. Knowing your zone will help you choose the right plants for your garden.

Our expert growers have created Growing Zone Guides for zones 4–9 in the United States, which span from Florida to Minnesota and coast to coast.

To find your zone, follow the instructions below:

1 Scan this QR code and enter your zip code.

2 Make note of your zone and turn to page 55 in our additional resources to find your Growing Zone Guide. These pages include a detailed list of the produce that thrives in your area and helpful tips based on your zone.

The Growing Zone Guide will provide you with a sample Garden Plan or help you customize your own. This plan has everything you need to select your seeds and create a planting and harvesting schedule.

When should I get started?

While preparations for planting begin in late winter or early spring, the main gardening season won't start until after the last spring frost.

🖉 **Turn to your Growing Zone Guide at the back of the book. Locate the date of the last frost and write it below. Then, set a planting date for yourself after the last frost and commit to playing in the dirt that day!**

DATE OF LAST FROST:

MY PLANTING DATE:

PREPARE

You've gotten your head in the gardening game. Now it's time to get your hands dirty! We've got two tasks for you to prepare your garden: Gather your supplies and build the bed.

Gather Your Supplies

Before you go shopping, take inventory of the supplies you already have (or the ones you can borrow). Check the boxes on your list as you find or purchase supplies!

GARDENING TOOLS

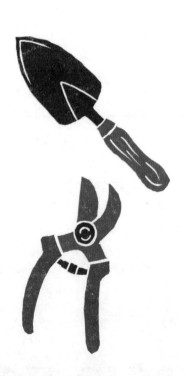

- ☐ **Hand tools:**
  - ‣ Hand trowel for digging
  - ‣ Hand rake for collecting debris and leaves
  - ‣ Hand hoe for weeding
  - ‣ Hand broom for cleaning off bed from compost
  - ‣ Hand fork to loosen soil
  - ‣ Hand cultivator to loosen soil and remove weeds
  - ‣ Pruning shears

- ☐ Plant labels
- ☐ Apron for holding tools and keeping your clothes clean
- ☐ A watering can

Scan this QR code to shop for supplies.

IF YOU'RE BUILDING A RAISED BED

- ☐ A box of 3-inch deck screws (you'll need around 100)
- ☐ A countersink drill bit (to pre-drill holes)
- ☐ A power drill

Lumber:

- ☐ **Six 8-foot boards** (2 inches wide, 10 inches high, 8 feet long)
  - ▸ Have the lumber store cut two of the boards in half.
  - ▸ Buy wood that hasn't been pressure treated or compressed. These woods contain chemicals that are harmful to the soil and your health.

- ☐ **Five two-by-fours** (2 inches wide, 4 inches high, 10 feet long)
  - ▸ Two of these will be used to make six support posts. Have the lumber store cut them into 18.5" pieces.
  - ▸ Three of these will be used to make the sitting ledges. Have the attendant cut one in half to make ledges for the 4-foot side. For the other two, have the attendant trim them down to 92 inches each.

NOTE: If you don't want to build a bed, we have raised bed kits for sale in our store. See the QR code on the previous page!

IF YOU'RE PLANTING DIRECTLY IN THE GROUND

- ☐ Hoe
- ☐ Cultivator/tiller
- ☐ Shovel
- ☐ Wheelbarrow

SEEDS AND SOIL

Once you decide which vegetables to put in your garden, order one packet of seeds per plant. (See your Growing Zone Guide at the back of the book for a list of options!)

- ☐ Seeds (one packet per crop)
- ☐ Soil
- ☐ Compost
- ☐ Mulch

SWAG

- ☐ Gloves
- ☐ Floppy hat (if you're into that)
- ☐ Shoes you don't mind getting dirty

NICE TO HAVE (BUT NOT NECESSARY)

- ☐ Insect netting
- ☐ Frost cloth
- ☐ Wire hoops
- ☐ Fertilizer
- ☐ Steel mesh (used underneath your raised bed to ensure that animals don't dig into it)

Understanding Soil and Compost

When choosing soil and compost, the options can quickly become overwhelming. To make things simple, here are a few key principles:

- **Topsoil** has aeration, meaning that water can easily pass through it and drain. Plant roots need oxygen to thrive, so compact soil is no good for gardening.

- **Compost** makes your plants happy by providing organic matter that slowly nourishes your crops over time. It also helps retain moisture in the soil after watering.

With that in mind, let's talk about how to fill your planting spaces. Many garden centers or online sources will immediately point you to a raised bed or planting mix. While these mixes prioritize drainage, they're usually lacking nutrients—especially by your second year of growing. Instead, we recommend using one of the following two options:

- A 50/50 blend of screened topsoil (processed through a mesh to remove debris) and high-quality compost.

- A 33/33/33 mix of screened topsoil, compost, and raised bed mix.

Either of these options will provide a high-quality garden bed, with plenty of nutrients, drainage, and aeration for your plant roots.

Soil and compost are the most expensive part of the garden, but also the most important! To save money, visit your local nursery to buy topsoil and compost in bulk. After purchasing your individual components, mix them together thoroughly before filling your garden bed.

Build the Bed

We get it—this part might seem tricky! Scan this QR code to see one of our expert Liberty Gardeners assemble a 4' x 8' raised bed and follow their step-by-step instructions.

Watch the tutorial!

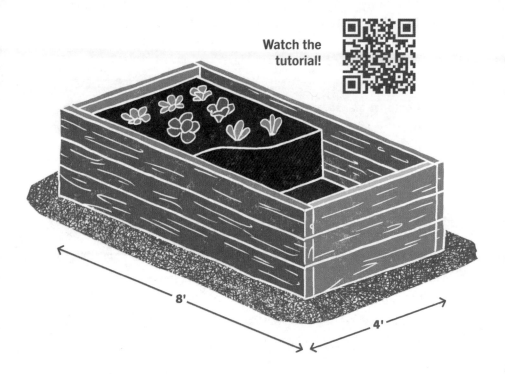

REMEMBER: You'll want to place your bed in a sunny part of your yard, with the 8-foot side running east to west for optimal sun exposure for your vegetables.

And if you want to skip the bed and plant directly into your soil, go for it! You'll need a good shovel to dig up the soil. Your cultivator and hoe can help, too. And we still recommend covering the top with high-quality soil and compost to give your plants lots of nutrients.

Filling the Bed with Soil

It's best to fill your garden bed to the top, because over the course of the year, the soil will settle and could end up 4–6 inches lower than the initial fill level.

Filling a raised bed requires quite a bit of volume. For example a 4' x 8' x 2' raised bed requires 64 cubic feet of material. This much soil can add up quickly. A great way to offset your cost is to fill the bottom 12 inches of your growing bed with whatever you have on hand: leaves, grass clippings, twigs, branches, or straw. But keep in mind that you need at least 12 inches of topsoil/compost for your crops to thrive.

Get a Head Start on Weed Prevention

After you've prepared your soil, cover it with cardboard until you're ready to plant. The cardboard will block sunlight and prevent weeds from taking up residence!

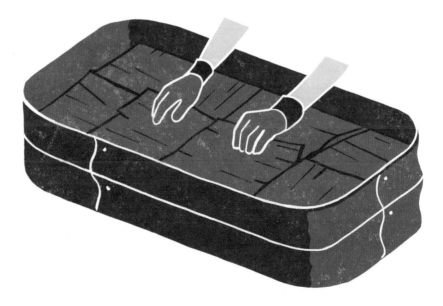

PLANT

It's finally here! Time to drop some seeds in the soil and step into your new life as a Liberty Gardener. Here's our go-to guide for planting your veggies.

REMEMBER: Most Crops Can't Handle Frost

Don't plant too early, or your seeds might not make it! Refer to the frost date in your Growing Zone Guide and follow your sample Garden Plan.

Give Your Seeds a Head Start

If you're eager to get growing, you can try **indoor seeding** for a majority of your vegetables. All you need is a few containers, your prepared soil/compost mixture, a south-facing window, and a willingness to bring dirt inside. Indoor seeding offers two main advantages: It protects fragile young seedlings from the unpredictable outdoors and it gives you a head start on your growing season.

For example, it takes broccoli 85 days to grow from seed to harvest. If you start inside instead of waiting for the great outdoors to heat up, you'll be able to produce a lot more broccoli over the season.

Want to give it a go? Refer to the Instructions for Indoor Seeding on page 106 to learn more.

Plant in 2' x 2' Squares

Put on your thinking cap. It's time for a little math.

Your 4' x 8' raised bed is designed to hold eight 2' x 2' plots. (If you're seeding directly into the ground instead of a raised bed, you can still use this layout to follow our growing plans.)

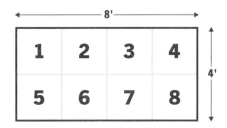

Using the sample Garden Plan from your Growing Zone Guide (or one you customized yourself), follow the template for planting in each plot. Refer to the spacing guide on page 92 to give your seeds plenty of breathing room.

Do You Have a Square to Spare?

Here's a gardening tip for parents of young kids. Getting your little ones involved in growing is an amazing experience, but it's not without its challenges. Sometimes kids cause unintentional damage to plants by being rough or harvesting early.

Try giving them their very own 2' x 2' plot to manage. They have full reign in their section, which means they need to let you have full reign in yours. You can still ask for their help with the rest of the garden, but giving them a section to manage is a great way to teach ownership while preserving most of the crop from overly eager tiny hands!

Prepare the Soil

If you haven't already, mix your topsoil and compost and place in your raised bed. Soil that's ready to seed needs to be loose—it should be easy to run your hand through it.

Use Your Finger (or a Trowel) to Dig the Holes

For small seeds, like lettuce and carrots, you can easily dig the shallow hole or row with your fingers. You might want to use a trowel to make holes for larger seeds (beans, peas, squash).

How deep should you dig? It depends on what you're planting. Follow the instructions on the back of each seed packet. These companies have done tons of research and know exactly what each seed needs.

Place the Seeds in the Holes

Following the instructions for spacing on page 92, place your seeds in their new home!

If you're planting directly in the soil, you'll want to overplant for your 2' x 2' plot, since some of your plants won't make it. Once your seeds have germinated (broken through the surface and sprouted), refer to the spacing guide and thin your seedlings, plucking out the necessary number to give the remaining plants plenty of space. Some plants—like arugula, mustard, and radishes—likely won't need to be thinned.

Gently Cover the Seeds with Soil

Use your hands to cover the seeds with just enough soil to make the holes even with the surface. Press down gently with your hand to make sure the seeds are in contact with the soil.

Label Your Rows

Use your bed labels to mark each 2' x 2' plot in your Liberty Garden. Write the name of the crop and the date you planted it.

"In the spring, at the end of the day, you should smell like dirt."

MARGARET ATWOOD

Give Your Seeds a Drink

To start the germination process (when a seed becomes a seedling), water the seeds *daily* with a watering can or hose with an adjustable nozzle. Make sure to use a gentle spray, not a strong stream of water that will wash the seeds away. Once they've germinated, you can reduce your watering according to the instructions in the Produce section of this guide.

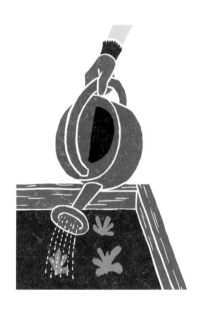

Cheers to Your Liberty Garden!

You did it! We hope there's lots of dirt under your nails and a smile on your face. You've made a very important step toward growing your own food. You've done the bulk of the work to get to this point, and now, the waiting begins.

Keep the Fun Going: Understanding Succession Planting

Seeding isn't a one-and-done process for your garden: You'll do this many more times this season to make the most of the spring, summer, and fall harvests.

Succession planting is a method that allows you to produce a continuous harvest of crops throughout the year. When one crop is harvested, use your sample Garden Plan to immediately plant another to maximize your space and create a continuous harvest. You don't want one of your 2' x 2' plots standing empty for long, so follow the timelines closely and replant as soon as a space opens up.

Strengthen Your Crops with Companion Planting

Companion planting is a gardening technique where different plants are grown close together for mutual benefit.

Companion planting helps keep pests away (like planting marigolds next to tomatoes) or improve the soil (like planting nitrogen-fixing beans next to corn). Some plants offer physical support to climbing plants, and others create helpful microclimates for shade-loving plants. Overall, companion planting makes crops stronger, healthier, and more balanced as they grow. It's a fascinating and beautiful phenomenon, just like nature intended.

On the flip side, some vegetables do not make for good companions. They compete for resources or produce chemicals that inhibit the other plant's growth. Here are a few combinations to avoid planting next to each other in your square plots:

▸ **Tomatoes and Potatoes:** Both are susceptible to similar pests and diseases, particularly blight, so it's best to plant them separately.

- **Cabbage and Strawberries:** Cabbage and other brassicas (like kale and broccoli) can release compounds that stunt the growth of strawberries.

- **Beans/Peas and Onions:** Onions release strong smells and chemicals that can hinder the growth of beans and peas. They can also compete for nutrients in the soil.

- **Corn and Tomatoes:** While these two plants thrive in similar conditions, corn can overshadow and shade tomatoes, limiting their sunlight. They can also attract the same type of pests.

- **Spinach and Potatoes:** Potatoes can shade spinach, preventing it from getting enough sunlight. And the shallow roots of spinach might compete with the deeper-rooting potatoes.

Three Sisters: Companion Planting at Its Finest

Native American tribes, especially the Iroquois and the Cherokee, developed a planting technique for the "Three Sisters": corn, beans, and squash. When grown close together, they support each other and create beautiful harmony. Corn provides a pole for beans to climb, beans enrich the soil with nitrogen, and squash spreads across the ground to retain moisture and prevent weeds. They also complement each other at harvest time, supplying carbohydrates, protein, and essential vitamins.

PRODUCE

From spring to fall, your goal as a Liberty Gardener is to create the ideal conditions for your crops to thrive. Start developing a habit of spending five minutes a day on three main tasks: watering, weeding, and warding off pests.

Watering Your Liberty Garden

There is no life without water. Follow these watering tips as you tend to your veggies:

▸ **Use a watering can or a hose with a nozzle.** You don't want to erode the soil with a heavy stream of water. Water the base of your plant to help it with absorption.

▸ **Be gentle with seedlings.** Starting out, your seedlings need frequent, light watering. The soil around them should stay moist, but don't overdo it.

▸ **Aim for 1–1.5 inches of water per week.** As your vegetables become more established, they need 1–1.5 inches of water per week—or about 20 gallons of water for your 4' x 8' bed. Plan to water your plants deeply about least twice a week (and adjust according to the guidelines on the next page).

> **"The best time to plant a tree was 20 years ago. The second best time is now."**

▸ **Check the moisture level before watering.** To see if your garden needs water, stick your finger in the dirt. If it's dry up to your knuckle, go for it! If it's moist, wait another day or two. You can also order a soil moisture meter for accurate readings.

▸ **Don't waterlog your plants.** Overwatering is bad for your crops! It can lead to root rot, fungus growth, and lack of oxygen by cutting off circulation in the soil. Plus, if your plants get too much water too frequently, they never develop strong root systems because they never have to dig deep in search of water.

▸ **Adjust according to your growing zone.** If you live in a hot, dry region, your plants will need more water. If you're in a cool or humid area where soil retains more moisture, you don't have to water as often.

▸ **Pay attention to the weather.** Sometimes, a nice rainfall will do your chores for you. Other times, in the hot summer months, your plants will get thirsty—so give them some extra love.

Weeding Your Liberty Garden

Where there is water and soil, weeds are sure to follow. The first step to dealing with weeds is to accept that they happen. Gardening is not a beauty contest. The goal is to grow healthy food and enjoy the process. Secondly, we understand how annoying they can be! But if you expect to encounter such nuisances, dealing with them becomes a lot easier.

Before we talk about how to manage weeds, we want to talk about how *not* to manage them: Please don't use harmful herbicides. They certainly get the job done, but they come with dangerous consequences to your health. Why grow healthy food if you're going to spray it with poison?

We cannot stress enough that Liberty Gardens Project is about flourishing. It's much better to have some weeds in your garden if it keeps toxic chemicals out of your body. When you commit to keeping toxins out of your garden, sometimes the weeds will win. And that's okay! Remember: Liberty Gardeners expect some failure with their crops. Everything is an experiment. Take joy in the learning process.

Eating Whole Foods the Way Nature Intended

Our grocery stores are full of GMO (genetically modified organism) foods. These plant and animal products are created from DNA altered in a lab using genetic engineering. These tweaks introduce traits like pest resistance, herbicide tolerance, or improved shelf life. While these "Frankenfoods," as some activists call them, can boost production and availability, studies have shown GMOs have a negative impact on the environment and on our bodies.

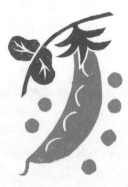

Your Liberty Garden offers an affordable way to eat non-GMO, organic whole foods—just like nature intended. Eating straight from your garden means fresher, nutrient-dense options, promoting health and sustainability—for you, your family, and the earth entrusted to you.

With these two techniques, you can keep the weeds at bay and enjoy a healthy crop:

1 **Hand-weed regularly.** It's easiest to remove weeds when they are young, so check for new weeds every time you make your five-minute visit to the garden. Using your hand or your trowel, dig under the surface and gently pull, making sure to get the entire root out of the ground to prevent further growth. It's helpful to weed after a decent rain, as the soft soil makes it easier to uproot the weeds.

2 **Use mulch.** Once your vegetables have broken through the surface, covering the soil around them with two to three inches of mulch helps prevent weed growth. Mulch also retains moisture for your plants, reducing the frequency of your watering and cutting down on your water bill. Mulch has the added benefit of breaking down slowly over time, adding organic matter to soil.

Which Mulch Should I Use?

When it comes to mulch, you've got options. Here are a few to consider:

▸ **Grass Clippings:** If your yard is free of fertilizers, pesticides, and weeds, you can mow it and spread your clippings in your garden as a mulch. Grass isn't a great mulch for fruiting plants (fruit plants, as well as tomatoes, peppers, cucumbers, and zucchini), however, because it's pure nitrogen, which slows the fruiting process. Also, only use grass clippings that are dry or only slightly damp. Wet grass will clump together, cutting off oxygen to the soil and, therefore, to your plants' roots.

- **Straw (Not Hay):** Straw is an excellent mulch due to being high in carbon. It also provides structure and doesn't blow around like grass. It breaks down slowly, adding nutrients to the soil over time. You can purchase straw from a local garden nursery, farm supply store, or perhaps directly from a farmer in your area. Make sure it does not contain seeds, as you don't want to introduce unwanted crops to your garden!

- **Fall Leaves:** In the later months of your growing season, rake the leaves in your yard and transfer some to your bed as mulch. As the leaves decompose, they release valuable nutrients, naturally fertilizing your soil and making an inviting space for earthworms. Shredding leaves (with a shredder, shears, or by mowing them and emptying the bag) before mulching helps them break down faster and prevents matting, which blocks airflow to the soil.

- **Wood Chips:** Blending large and small wood chips with shredded leaves creates an ecosystem similar to a forest floor, where weeds don't grow. Fresh wood chips are pure carbon, which extracts nitrogen from the soil, so it's better to use aged wood chips. You can purchase them from a farm supply or home improvement store. At the end of the season, don't mix the chips into the soil—the high amount of carbon will steal nutrients.

- **Synthetic Fabric:** One other approach is to cover the soil around your plants with synthetic fabric, which you can purchase at a local gardening center. Make sure to cut holes for your plants to grow through! The fabric is porous, allowing water through for your plants while blocking and killing seeds.

Warding Off Pests

Weeds aren't the only threats to your garden—you also need to keep an eye out for pests. Again, we urge you to commit to a toxin-free approach. Here are a few alternative ways to protect your garden:

Spot the symptoms. Noticing pests early on will help you get a jump start on prevention. Here are signs that pests may be wreaking havoc on your plants:

- Tiny dots on leaves
- Webs on plants
- Holes in leaves or vegetables
- Wilting or stunted plants
- Curled leaves
- Yellowing leaves
- Decay

Look for these common pests. While are there are quite literally hundreds of potential pests, here are a few of the most common, along with a description of the damage they cause:

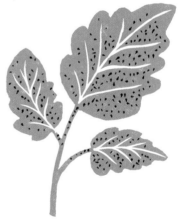

- **Aphids:** These small, soft-bodied insects can be green, black, or brown. They suck sap from plants, leading to stunted growth, curled leaves, and a sticky residue called honeydew.

- **Spider Mites:** These tiny, spider-like pests are often found on the undersides of leaves. They feed on plant sap, causing leaves to turn yellow and look covered in dots. Since they're spiders, they also leave their webbing on plants.

- **Whiteflies:** These small, white, winged insects resemble tiny moths. They feed on the undersides of leaves, leading to yellowing, wilting, and potential diseases.

- **Slugs and Snails:** These familiar soft and slimy crawlers leave a shiny trail wherever they go. They chew irregular holes in leaves, stems, and fruits.

- **Caterpillars:** The larval stage of moths and butterflies, these common pests are often green or brown. They can cause significant damage by chewing large holes in leaves and sometimes feeding on fruits and flowers.

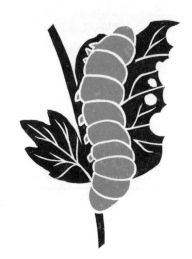

- **Japanese Beetles:** These metallic green and bronze beetles feed on leaves, flowers and fruits.

"You know that the beginning is the most important part of any work, especially in the case of a young and tender thing."

PLATO

Set up a fence to keep larger animals out. You're not the only one excited about your tasty vegetables: Deer, rabbits, raccoons, groundhogs, skunks, and squirrels might also try to get a bite! If you're having issues with larger animals, you might consider building a fence around your garden, covering the plants with nets, or planting some strong-smelling herbs, which act as deterrents.

Maintain nutritious soil. Insects attack weak plants, and plants become weak when they don't have the nutrients they need in the soil. Think of your soil like keeping a full bank account. Every time a withdrawal is made (i.e. plants eat up the nutrients), you need to make a deposit. Adding compost to your soil every spring and organic fertilizer before every crop will help keep your soil rich. You can purchase fertilizer at a garden store and follow the instructions on the bag.

Try a natural spray. We recommend a few pesticides that won't cause you or your family harm: Neem Oil, Diatomaceous Earth, and Insecticidal Soap. But use them intentionally, only targeting affected plants, as they can also kill beneficial insects.

Use your hands. The small scale of a Liberty Garden makes it possible to pick pests by hand. Use your gardening gloves to protect yourself from bites or stings.

Get some beer and duct tape. No, this isn't a lyric to a country song. With a little bit of research, you can find all sorts of hacks to prevent specific pests. For example, slugs and snails are attracted to the scent of beer. If they're giving you trouble, place a shallow dish of beer in your garden. The slugs and snails will make their way to it and drown (RIP). Duct tape acts as a nontoxic trap for pests—much like a sticky fly trap. Lay strips of tape around the affected plants or hang them up from stakes in the ground. Use brightly colored tape to attract the bugs even more.

PARTAKE

And now, the moment you've been waiting for! Whether it's the orange hint of a carrot peeking through the dirt or a ripe red tomato ready to fall off the vine, seeing your hard-earned vegetables at their peak—ready to be savored—is indeed a moment of joy.

To partake with the utmost enjoyment, here are a few guidelines for harvesting your vegetables.

> ## "Eat deliberately, with other people whenever possible, and always with pleasure."
>
> **MICHAEL POLLAN**

Tips for a Prosperous Harvest

While every vegetable has nuanced needs for harvesting, here are a few general guidelines that will help you pick your plants at the right time.

Wait Until They're Ready

In each Growing Zone Guide, we've provided a sample Garden Plan for you to follow, with a date range for harvesting. Follow that guide closely, check your vegetables regularly for signs of ripeness, and use your common sense.

Also, exercise patience! Sometimes, vegetables look good—and they might be edible—but they haven't reached their full potential. For example, a head of lettuce may look ready to harvest at 40 days, but in the next 20 days, it becomes more dense and tightened up, just like you'll see with store-bought lettuce. If you want full, mature, delicious lettuce, you have to wait the full 60 days.

Take Care When Cutting Your Crops

Morning is ideal for harvesting, since the plants are crisp and hydrated. Some veggies can be simply pulled out of the earth or gently coaxed from the stem (like carrots or tomatoes).

But as you harvest crops that need to be cut from their plant—lettuce, broccoli, kale, zucchini, and more—use a sharp, non-serrated knife. Serrated knives cut your greens in multiple spots and damage them. We recommend the Opinel (non-serrated) gardening knife or a Victorinox (non-serrated) knife.

Wash Your Veggies Thoroughly

To avoid cross contamination, follow these tips for washing your vegetables:

- ▸ Clean your washing area (sink, bowls, etc.) before beginning.
- ▸ Wash your hands first to avoid transferring bacteria to the plants.
- ▸ Thoroughly rinse your vegetables in cold running water to remove dirt.
- ▸ Use a vegetable brush for firmer produce, like sweet potatoes and squash.
- ▸ Allow your vegetables to dry completely before storing (removing excess water helps prevent bacterial growth).

PRO TIP: Wait to wash your vegetables until you are ready to eat, can, or freeze them. Leaving them dirty helps them store for longer periods!

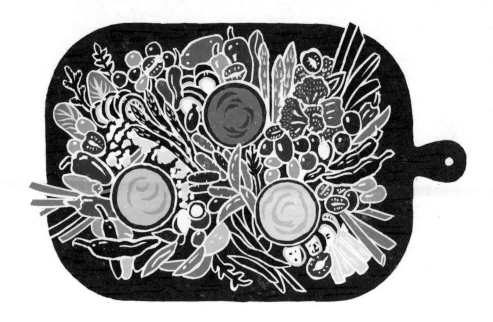

Bon Appétit!

At Liberty Gardens Project, we believe the best part of growing food isn't the food itself—it's the invitation to a flourishing life. There's nothing better than enjoying food you love with people you love even more. After all, veggies taste best when shared.

You should feel proud of the work you've done and be ready to celebrate! Find a way to pause and savor your incredible accomplishment—whether that's by inviting a few friends over for a harvest party, chopping up fresh veggies to serve to your kids, or incorporating your homegrown food into your own dinner.

A garden teaches us that more is always possible. Armed with seeds and soil, we find an endless supply of abundance and an expectation for good things to come in the future.

Cheers to the flourishing life!

ADDITIONAL RESOURCES

Our team at Liberty Gardens Project has
put together a video library of tutorials.

Scan this QR code to learn tips on
planting, watering, harvesting, and more!

PREPARING FOR NEXT YEAR

Life picks up in the fall. Before you know it, the holidays will fly by and you'll be welcoming a new year. As you wrap up your growing season, work through this checklist to get a head start on next year's garden.

- ☐ **Get rid of all weeds.** Thoroughly weed your garden and remove all diseased plants. You can uproot healthy plants and leave them in the garden soil to compost.

- ☐ **Add compost.** Add a layer of compost to your garden bed to enrich it for next year. Mix it into your existing soil.

- ☐ **Mulch.** Add mulch to retain moisture and prevent weeds from taking over.

- ☐ **Cover your garden for the winter months.** Cover your garden with plastic sheets or frost cloths. This helps create a warm greenhouse effect and kills early weeds. It's also a great environment for earthworms to burrow, breaking down the compost you've added and creating loose, airy soil.

- ☐ **Put away your garden tools.** Clean your tools, remove all dirt, and store them for next year. Consider sharpening tools that need it so they're ready to go in the spring.

- ☐ **Reflect on this growing season.** Using the prompts on the next two pages, think about what you learned this year and plan your next season.

Garden Notes

✏️ What went well this year? What were some wins for you and your garden?

....

....

....

✏️ How did it feel to grow your own food?

....

....

....

✏️ What challenges did you face in your garden this year? What resources could help you overcome them next year?

....

....

....

....

....

✏️ **What would you like to grow again? What different crops would you like to try next year?**

....

....

....

✏️ **In the space below, jot down any lessons you learned—about gardening or life—through this experience.**

....

....

....

....

....

....

....

....

....

GROWING ZONE GUIDES

If you haven't already figured out your growing zone, scan this QR code and enter your zip code:

USDA Plant Hardiness Zone Map

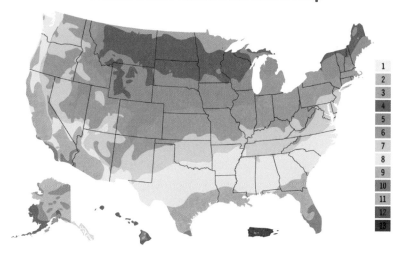

A quick note of explanation: While the USDA's map divides zones into "a" and "b," (for example, zone 7a and zone 7b), our Liberty Gardens Growing Zone Guides combine the two. The differences are too nuanced to affect beginning gardeners.

The most important piece of information on your Growing Zone Guide is the frost date. In the spring, you don't want to plant or transplant before that date, or else your tender seedlings may not make it. In the fall, you want to harvest most veggies before the frost date (some, like kale, can withstand the cold).

GROWING ZONE 4

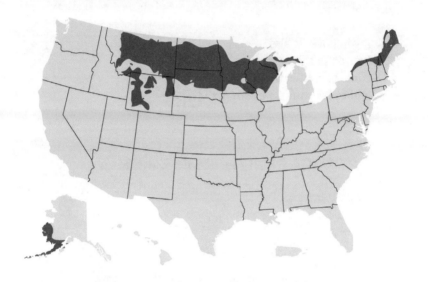

Summary: Growing zone 4 is characterized by having a climate with cold winters and moderate summers. It's more challenging to grow vegetables in this zone, as compared to other regions, yet it's ideal for hardy plants. Typical annual minimum temperatures in winter months range from -30ºF to -20ºF and average annual highs in summer months range from 60ºF to 75ºF. Rainfall in growing zone 4 can vary dramatically depending on the growing location—averaging 12–40 inches annually.

Frost: Zone 4 has one of the shortest growing seasons in the U.S., with only 90–120 frost-free growing days. Frost in this growing zone is going to be heavily impacted by altitude, proximity to water, and number of windbreaks (trees, shrubs, fence lines—anything that reduces wind).

- **Last (spring) frost:** Late May to early June
- **First (fall) frost:** Late September to early October

Zone 4 Tips

- **Increase growing space.** Because the growing season in zone 4 is so short, increasing your number of beds will allow you to grow more plants during the season.

- **Transplant as much and as late as possible.** Starting seeds inside will help you make the most of your harvest. By getting a head start and setting out full-sized plants, you'll likely be able to get two crops in the bed across the season or have a full yield of tomatoes!

- **Use plastic covers for hot weather crops.** Using greenhouse plastic and hoops over crops like tomatoes, peppers, eggplants, melons, and winter squash during the beginning of their growth will give them a head start and allow for quicker time to maturity.

- **Pay attention to watering needs.** Watering in dry regions can be difficult since you're not getting help from rainfall. However, dryland vegetables have a rich, concentrated flavor because they have less water concentration in the fruit. So putting in the work is worth it! Vegetables typically need 1 inch of water per week, so a 4' x 8' garden bed across 16 weeks of growing will require around 260 gallons of water throughout the season. Make sure you have a good watering system in place—whether that's a hose or a watering can. Also, adding organic matter like compost to your soil helps it retain moisture.

Plan Ahead with Your Crop Calendar

Turn the page to see your zone's crop calendar—the master list of when each vegetable should be planted and harvested, according to your frost dates. We've broken the two pages into the spring/summer and the fall seasons to make it easier to read.

ZONE 4	SPRING / SUMMER			
Crop	Indoor Seeding	Outdoor Seeding	Transplanting	Harvest
Arugula		4/10–7/5		5/15–8/5
Basil	3/20–7/20	5/15–7/20	5/15–8/20	6/15–9/25
Beans		5/7–7/15		7/5–9/20
Beets	3/15–4/15	4/15–5/15	4/15–5/15	6/20–7/15
Bok Choy				
Broccoli	3/7–4/15	4/2–4/9	4/15–5/15	6/1–7/5
Brussels Sprouts		5/15–6/1		9/1–10/1
Cabbage	3/7–4/15	4/2–4/9	4/15–5/15	6/1–7/5
Carrots		4/10–8/1		6/15–10/25
Cauliflower	3/7–4/15	4/2–4/9	4/15–5/15	6/1–7/5
Chard	3/15–4/15	4/15–5/15	4/15–5/15	6/20–7/15
Chicory	3/28–6/1	4/15–7/1	4/20–7/1	5/20–8/1
Corn		5/15–6/25		8/1–9/10
Cucumbers	4/15–6/30	5/15–7/1	5/15–7/30	7/10–9/25
Eggplant	3/20–6/10		5/15–7/20	7/25–9/25
Fennel	3/20–6/15	5/10–6/15	4/20–7/15	6/20–9/20
Garlic				
Green Onions	3/1–4/15	4/15–5/15	4/15–5/15	6/20–7/15
Kale	3/10–4/20	4/20–5/20	4/20–5/20	5/20–7/20
Leeks	3/1–4/20		4/20–6/1	7/15–9/15
Lettuce	3/28–6/1	4/15–7/1	4/20–7/1	5/20–8/1
Melons	4/20–6/1	5/20–6/15	5/20–7/1	7/25–9/25
Mustard		4/10–7/5		5/15–8/5
Okra	4/10–5/15	5/20–6/5	5/15–7/20	7/25–9/25
Onions	3/1–4/20		4/20–6/1	7/15–9/15
Peppers	3/20–6/10		5/15–7/20	7/25–9/25
Peas		4/10–5/30		6/10–8/1
Potatoes		4/10–5/15		7/1–8/20
Radishes		4/10–7/5		5/15–8/5
Spinach	3/15–6/1	4/10–6/1	4/15–7/1	5/20–8/1
Strawberries			5/1–6/1	8/1–9/1
Summer Squash/Zucchini	4/20–7/1	5/20–6/25	5/20–7/25	6/25–9/25
Sweet Potatoes			5/20–6/20	8/20–9/20
Tomatoes	3/20–6/10		5/15–7/20	7/25–9/25
Turnips		4/10–6/1		5/25–7/15
Winter Squash/Pumpkins	4/25–6/1	5/20–6/15	5/20–6/15	7/25–9/15

ZONE 4	FALL			
Crop	Indoor Seeding	Outdoor Seeding	Transplanting	Harvest
Arugula		7/10–9/10		8/10–10/20
Basil				
Beans				
Beets	6/15–8/1	7/15–8/1	7/15–9/1	8/5–10/5
Bok Choy				
Broccoli	6/25–7/5	7/5–7/15	7/25–8/5	9/1–10/20
Brussels Sprouts				
Cabbage	6/25–7/5	7/5–7/15	7/25–8/5	9/1–10/20
Carrots				
Cauliflower	6/25–7/5	7/5–7/15	7/25–8/5	9/1–10/20
Chard	6/15–8/10	7/15–8/15	7/15–9/10	8/5–10/5
Chicory	7/5–8/5	7/5–8/1	8/5–9/5	9/5–10/5
Corn				
Cucumbers				
Eggplant				
Fennel				
Garlic		10/10–11/3		7/10–8/15
Green Onions	6/10–8/1	7/15–8/1	7/15–9/1	8/5–10/5
Kale	6/20–7/5	7/20–8/5	7/20–8/5	8/20–10/5
Leeks				
Lettuce	7/5–8/5	7/5–8/1	8/5–9/5	9/5–11/1
Melons				
Mustard		7/10–9/10		8/10–10/20
Okra				
Onions				
Peppers				
Peas		6/10–7/15		8/10–9/15
Potatoes				
Radishes		7/10–9/10		8/10–10/20
Spinach	6/5–8/1	6/5–8/15	7/5–9/5	8/5–10/20
Strawberries				
Summer Squash/Zucchini				
Sweet Potatoes				
Tomatoes				
Turnips		6/5–8/15		7/20–10/1
Winter Squash/Pumpkins				

ZONE 4
GARDEN PLAN

To make your first Liberty Garden as simple as possible, we've put together a sample Garden Plan that will guide you every step of the way.

The numbers 1–8 represent the 2' x 2' square plots. You'll plant one vegetable in each. Follow along at the top of the Garden Plan to know what to do each month.

Along the timelines, you'll notice a few key instructions:

S - Ready to Seed
H - Time to Harvest

These instructions are for outdoor seeding only. If you want to seed indoors and transplant (T) to your garden, reference pages 106–107 and adjust your dates accordingly.

Scan the QR code to download a PDF of your sample Garden Plan. You can keep a copy on the fridge or wherever you keep your gardening supplies.

SAMPLE GARDEN PLAN – ZONE 4

S = Seed   H = Harvest   T = Recommended to Seed Indoors and Transplant

GARDEN BOXES	Planting schedule (months JAN–DEC, weeks 1–4)
1	**Carrots** — S (Apr) … H S (Jun) · **Summer Squash (T)** … H (Sep)
2	**Peppers (T)** — S Lettuce (T) H S (Apr–May) … H S Lettuce (T) H (Aug–Sep)
3	**Radishes** S … H (Apr–May) · **Cucumbers** S … H S · **Spinach (T)** … H (Oct)
4	**Arugula** S … H (May) · **Tomatoes (T)** S … H (Sep)
5	**Broccoli (T)** S … H S (Jun) · **Melons (T)** … H (Sep)
6	**Potatoes** S … S (Aug) · **Kale (T)** … H (Oct)
7	**Onions** S … H S · **Carrots** … H (Oct)
8	**Beets** S … H S (Jun) · **Corn** … H S **Radishes** H (Sep–Oct)

MONTH: JAN · FEB · MAR · APR · MAY · JUN · JUL · AUG · SEP · OCT · NOV · DEC
WEEKS: 1 2 3 4 (per month)

Legend key blocks: 1 2 3 4 / 5 6 7 8

GROWING ZONE 5

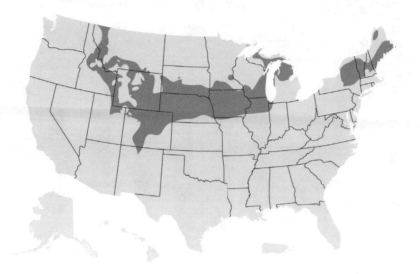

Summary: Growing zone 5 is characterized by cold winters and mild, enjoyable summers. Growing zone 5 is conducive to a wide range of gardening possibilities. Annual minimum temperatures in winter months typically range from -20ºF to -10ºF and average annual highs in summer months range from 60ºF to 80ºF. Rainfall in growing zone 5 averages 25–40 inches per year; however, in some dry regions of zone 5, rainfall can fall below 25 inches per year.

Frost: Zone 5 has 143–180 frost-free growing days, making the success rate for almost all annual vegetables very high. The high number of chill days (under 32ºF) make zone 5 one of the best fruit growing regions in the United States (consider growing strawberries, blackberries, or raspberries in your Liberty Garden)!

- ▸ **Last (spring) frost:** May 1 to May 15
- ▸ **First (fall) frost:** October 5 to October 20

Zone 5 Tips

▸ **Start your seeds inside and transplant.** Starting seeds inside will help you make the most of your harvest. By getting a head start and setting out full-sized plants, you'll likely be able to get two crops in the bed across the season or have a full yield of tomatoes!

▸ **Cover your crops with frost cloth.** Frost cloth (with hoops for support) can be placed over vegetables in the spring or fall when there is a potential for frost overnight. The frost cloth will keep the vegetables 3–4º warmer than the outside temperatures and safe from the wind, which is the real killer!

▸ **Use plastic covers for hot weather crops.** Using greenhouse plastic and hoops over crops like tomatoes, peppers, eggplants, melons, and winter squash during the beginning of their growth will give them a head start and allow for quicker time to maturity.

▸ **Use straw mulch strategically.** Avoid straw mulch early in the season because it will trap cold air in the soil when the soil needs to be heating up. However, using straw in the summer helps retain moisture and avoids high temperature fluctuations between night and day. Use straw until plants are established (around four to six weeks old).

Plan Ahead with Your Crop Calendar

Turn the page to see your zone's crop calendar—the master list of when each vegetable should be planted and harvested, according to your frost dates. We've broken the two pages into the spring/summer and the fall seasons to make it easier to read.

ZONE 5	SPRING / SUMMER			
Crop	Indoor Seeding	Outdoor Seeding	Transplanting	Harvest
Arugula		3/25–6/25		4/25–7/25
Basil	4/10–7/1	5/10–8/1	5/10–8/1	5/25–10/5
Beans		5/1–7/25		6/25–10/1
Beets	3/10–4/10	4/10–5/10	4/10–5/10	5/10–7/10
Bok Choy	3/10–5/1	5/5–5/15	4/10–5/25	5/5–7/1
Broccoli	2/25–4/7	4/10–4/25	4/10–5/7	5/20–6/25
Brussels Sprouts	5/1–7/1	5/1–7/1	6/1–8/1	9/1–11/1
Cabbage	2/25–4/7	4/10–4/25	4/10–5/7	5/20–6/25
Carrots		3/25–8/5		6/1–10/21
Cauliflower	2/25–4/7	4/10–4/25	4/10–5/7	5/20–6/25
Chard	3/15–4/1	4/5–4/25	4/10–5/1	5/5–7/5
Chicory	3/15–5/15	4/10–5/15	4/10–6/15	5/15–7/15
Corn		5/8–7/15		7/20–9/25
Cucumbers	4/5–7/5	5/8–7/15	5/8–8/1	6/5–10/5
Eggplant	3/15–6/15	5/20–6/5	5/15–7/15	7/20–10/1
Fennel	3/15–4/1	5/1–5/10	4/25–5/10	6/1–8/10
Garlic				
Green Onions	2/25–4/15	4/15–6/1	4/15–6/1	6/1–7/25
Kale	2/25–4/10	4/10–4/20	3/25–5/10	5/10–7/10
Leeks	2/10–3/1		4/2–4/20	6/10–8/1
Lettuce	3/15–5/15	4/5–6/1	4/5–6/15	5/5–8/1
Melons	4/10–6/15	5/1–6/15	5/10–7/15	7/15–10/1
Mustard		3/25–6/25		4/25–7/25
Okra		5/10–7/5		7/25–10/1
Onions	2/20–3/10	3/15–4/10	4/1–5/15	7/30–9/20
Peppers	3/15–6/15	5/20–6/5	5/15–7/15	7/20–10/1
Peas		3/25–5/10		5/25–7/10
Potatoes		3/25–4/15		6/20–8/15
Radishes		3/25–6/25		4/25–7/25
Spinach	2/20–5/15	3/25–5/8	3/22–6/5	4/20–7/30
Strawberries			4/5–5/1	6/15–7/20
Summer Squash/Zucchini	4/10–7/1	5/10–7/5	5/10–8/1	6/25–10/1
Sweet Potatoes			5/10–7/1	9/10–10/10
Tomatoes	3/15–6/15	5/20–6/5	5/15–7/15	7/20–10/1
Turnips		3/25–6/25		5/15–8/15
Winter Squash/Pumpkins	4/5–7/5	5/8–7/5	5/8–8/1	9/1–10/30

ZONE 5	FALL			
Crop	Indoor Seeding	Outdoor Seeding	Transplanting	Harvest
Arugula		7/25–9/15		8/25–10/15
Basil				
Beans				
Beets	7/20–8/20	7/20–8/20	8/20–9/20	9/20–10/20
Bok Choy	7/10–8/15	8/5–9/1	8/10–9/15	9/1–10/15
Broccoli	7/5–7/20	7/15–7/22	8/5–8/20	9/5–10/25
Brussels Sprouts				
Cabbage	7/5–7/20	7/15–7/22	8/5–8/20	9/5–10/25
Carrots				
Cauliflower	7/5–7/20	7/15–7/22	8/5–8/20	9/5–10/25
Chard	7/15–8/1	8/1–8/20	8/15–9/1	10/1–11/1
Chicory	7/15–8/15	8/15–9/1	8/15–9/15	9/20–11/1
Corn				
Cucumbers				
Eggplant				
Fennel	7/5–8/1	7/15–8/1	8/5–9/1	9/5–10/1
Garlic		10/20–11/10		7/1–8/1
Green Onions	6/25–8/1	6/25–8/1	7/15–9/15	9/1–10/25
Kale	7/5–8/1	8/5–8/20	8/5–9/1	9/15–11/15
Leeks				
Lettuce	7/15–8/5	8/5–8/20	8/15–9/5	9/15–10/5
Melons				
Mustard		7/25–9/15		8/25–10/15
Okra				
Onions				
Peppers				
Peas		7/15–8/1		9/15–10/15
Potatoes				
Radishes		7/25–9/15		8/25–10/15
Spinach	7/15–8/20	8/15–9/15	8/15–9/25	9/10–12/1
Strawberries				
Summer Squash/Zucchini				
Sweet Potatoes				
Tomatoes				
Turnips		8/1–9/15		9/20–10/20
Winter Squash/Pumpkins				

ZONE 5
GARDEN PLAN

To make your first Liberty Garden as simple as possible, we've put together a sample Garden Plan that will guide you every step of the way.

The numbers 1—8 represent the 2' x 2' square plots. You'll plant one vegetable in each. Follow along at the top of the Garden Plan to know what to do each month.

Along the timelines, you'll notice a few key instructions:

S - Ready to Seed
H - Time to Harvest

These instructions are for outdoor seeding only. If you want to seed indoors and transplant (T) to your garden, reference pages 106—107 and adjust your dates accordingly.

Scan the QR code to download a PDF of your sample Garden Plan. You can keep a copy on the fridge or wherever you keep your gardening supplies.

SAMPLE GARDEN PLAN - ZONE 5

S = Seed   H = Harvest   T = Recommended to Seed Indoors and Transplant

	1	2	3	4
	5	6	7	8

GARDEN BOXES

Box 1: S Carrots H S Peppers (T) H

Box 2: S Lettuce (T) H S Summer Squash (T) H Carrots H

Box 3: S Radishes H S Cucumbers H Beets H

Box 4: S Arugula H S Broccoli (T) S Tomatoes (T) H S Spinach (T) H

Box 5: S Broccoli (T) H S Corn H S Lettuce (T) H

Box 6: S Potatoes S Kale (T) H

Box 7: S Onions H S Basil (T) H S Arugula H

Box 8: S Beets H S Melons (T) H S Radishes H

MONTH / WEEKS: JAN 1 2 3 4 · FEB 1 2 3 4 · MAR 1 2 3 4 · APR 1 2 3 4 · MAY 1 2 3 4 · JUN 1 2 3 4 · JUL 1 2 3 4 · AUG 1 2 3 4 · SEP 1 2 3 4 · OCT 1 2 3 4 · NOV 1 2 3 4 · DEC 1 2 3 4

GROWING ZONE 6

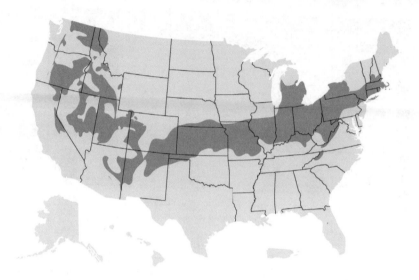

Summary: Growing zone 6 has a moderate climate with mild winters and warm summers, making it perfect for gardening! Annual minimum temperatures in winter months typically range from -10ºF to 0ºF and annual high temperatures during the summer months typically range from 65ºF to 85ºF. Rainfall in growing zone 6 averages 30–50 inches per year. However, dry and mountainous regions in zone 6 can expect far less than average rainfall.

Frost: Zone 6 is one of the best growing zones in the country for annual crops, boasting 180–210 frost-free days. Growing zone 6 also has enough chill days (under 32ºF) to grow fruit very successfully.

- **Last (spring) frost:** April 1 to April 20
- **First (fall) frost:** October 13 to October 31

Zone 6 Tips

- **Cover your crops with frost cloth.** Frost cloth (with hoops for support) can be placed over vegetables in the spring or fall when there is a potential for frost overnight. The frost cloth will keep the vegetables 3–4º warmer than the outside temperatures and safe from the wind, which is the real killer!

- **Start seeds indoors or plant directly in the ground.** The longer growing time in zone 6 gives you time to plant seeds directly in the dirt and get a second crop in before the end of the season. However, if you choose to seed indoors and transplant your crops, there's a potential to get three crops in the same garden bed throughout the season!

- **Retain moisture through mulching.** Mulching a garden bed with straw or wood chips can retain moisture throughout the season. But do not mix the mulch into the soil once the crop is done growing. The mulch will bond with nitrogen in the soil and reduce the soil fertility over time.

- **Plant successions.** Succession planting allows you to have a continuous harvest of one crop throughout the year. For example, in growing zone 6 you could enjoy tomatoes from July to October. Plant a tomato plant every four weeks (for example in late April, late May, and late June) to harvest tomatoes all season long.

Plan Ahead with Your Crop Calendar

Turn the page to see your zone's crop calendar—the master list of when each vegetable should be planted and harvested, according to your frost dates. We've broken the two pages into the spring/summer and the fall seasons to make it easier to read.

ZONE 6	SPRING / SUMMER			
Crop	Indoor Seeding	Outdoor Seeding	Transplanting	Harvest
Arugula		3/7–6/7		4/10–7/7
Basil	4/1–7/5	5/1–8/5	5/20–8/5	6/25–10/10
Beans		4/20–8/5		8/15–10/5
Beets	3/1–4/15	4/1–5/15	4/1–5/15	5/20–7/1
Bok Choy	3/1–4/20	4/1–5/7	4/1–5/20	5/5–6/20
Broccoli	2/20–4/1	4/1–5/1	4/1–5/1	5/15–6/20
Brussels Sprouts	5/1–7/15	5/1–7/15	6/1–8/15	9/1–11/15
Cabbage	2/20–4/1	4/1–5/1	4/1–5/1	5/15–6/20
Carrots		3/15–6/10		6/10–8/20
Cauliflower	2/20–4/1	4/1–5/1	4/1–5/1	5/15–6/20
Chard	3/5–4/1	4/2–4/30	4/5–5/1	4/29–7/5
Chicory	3/5–5/15	4/10–5/15	3/25–6/15	5/15–7/15
Corn		5/1–8/1		7/15–10/15
Cucumbers	3/25–7/15	4/30–7/10	4/25–8/15	5/20–10/10
Eggplant	3/1–7/1	5/15–6/15	5/10–8/1	7/15–10/20
Fennel	3/1–4/1	4/20–5/1	4/15–5/1	5/15–8/1
Garlic				
Green Onions	2/20–4/15	4/15–6/1	4/15–6/1	6/1–7/25
Kale	2/20–3/30	4/5–4/20	3/20–4/30	5/5–7/1
Leeks	2/5–2/20		3/25–4/10	7/25–8/15
Lettuce	3/1–5/15	4/1–5/15	3/25–6/5	5/5–7/5
Melons	4/1–6/20	4/25–7/1	4/25–7/20	7/10–10/5
Mustard		3/7–6/7		4/10–7/7
Okra		5/5–7/10		7/20–10/20
Onions	2/5–3/1	3/15–4/1	3/25–4/25	7/25–9/15
Peppers	3/1–7/1	5/15–6/15	5/10–8/1	7/15–10/10
Peas		3/15–5/1		5/15–7/15
Potatoes		3/15–4/10		6/20–8/1
Radishes		3/7–6/7		4/10–7/7
Spinach	2/20–4/15	3/25–5/1	3/15–5/15	4/20–7/1
Strawberries			4/1–5/1	6/15–7/20
Summer Squash/Zucchini	4/7–7/10	5/7–7/7	5/7–8/1	6/25–10/1
Sweet Potatoes		5/20–6/15		8/25–10/15
Tomatoes	3/1–7/1	5/15–6/15	5/10–8/1	7/15–10/10
Turnips		3/15–6/15		5/1–8/1
Winter Squash/Pumpkins	4/1–7/5	5/1–7/5	5/1–8/1	9/1–10/30

ZONE 6	FALL			
Crop	Indoor Seeding	Outdoor Seeding	Transplanting	Harvest
Arugula		8/15–10/1		9/15–11/1
Basil				
Beans				
Beets	7/15–8/15	7/25–8/26	8/15–9/15	9/15–10/15
Bok Choy	7/20–9/1	8/15–9/5	8/20–10/1	9/20–11/1
Broccoli	7/12–7/30	7/22–7/30	8/12–8/30	9/15–11/1
Brussels Sprouts				
Cabbage	7/12–7/30	7/22–7/30	8/12–8/30	9/15–11/1
Carrots		8/1–9/15		10/10–11/15
Cauliflower	7/12–7/30	7/22–7/30	8/12–8/30	9/15–11/1
Chard	7/15–8/15	8/10–9/1	8/15–9/15	9/15–11/10
Chicory	7/15–8/15	8/15–9/1	8/15–9/15	9/20–11/15
Corn				
Cucumbers				
Eggplant				
Fennel	7/10–8/5	7/20–8/5	8/10–9/1	9/15–10/10
Garlic		10/20–11/20		6/15–7/15
Green Onions	6/25–8/1	6/25–8/1	7/15–9/15	9/1–10/25
Kale	7/20–8/15	8/15–9/1	8/20–9/15	10/1–11/25
Leeks				
Lettuce	7/20–9/1	8/15–9/1	8/20–10/1	9/20–11/25
Melons				
Mustard		8/15–10/1		9/15–11/1
Okra				
Onions				
Peppers				
Peas		8/1–8/15		10/1–11/1
Potatoes				
Radishes		8/15–10/1		9/15–11/1
Spinach	7/15–9/1	8/15–9/15	8/15–10/1	9/10–12/1
Strawberries				
Summer Squash/Zucchini				
Sweet Potatoes				
Tomatoes				
Turnips		8/10–9/1		9/20–10/20
Winter Squash/Pumpkins				

ZONE 6
GARDEN PLAN

To make your first Liberty Garden as simple as possible, we've put together a sample Garden Plan that will guide you every step of the way.

The numbers 1—8 represent the 2' x 2' square plots. You'll plant one vegetable in each. Follow along at the top of the Garden Plan to know what to do each month.

Along the timelines, you'll notice a few key instructions:

S - Ready to Seed
H - Time to Harvest

These instructions are for outdoor seeding only. If you want to seed indoors and transplant (T) to your garden, reference pages 106—107 and adjust your dates accordingly.

Scan the QR code to download a PDF of your sample Garden Plan. You can keep a copy on the fridge or wherever you keep your gardening supplies.

SAMPLE GARDEN PLAN - ZONE 6

S = Seed   H = Harvest   T = Recommended to Seed Indoors and Transplant

GARDEN BOX	Crops (Seed → Harvest timeline)
1	Carrots (S Mar – H Jun); Peppers (T) (S Jun – H Sep)
2	Lettuce (T) (S Apr – H Apr); Summer Squash (T) (S May – H Jul); Carrots (S Jul – H Oct)
3	Radishes (S Mar – H Apr); Cucumbers (S May – H Jul); Beets (S Aug – H Oct)
4	Arugula (S Mar – H Apr); Tomatoes (T) (S May – H Sep); Arugula (S Sep – H Oct)
5	Broccoli (T) (S Mar – H Jun); Corn (S Jun – H Aug); Lettuce (T) (S Sep – H Oct)
6	Potatoes (S Mar – H Jun); Basil (T) (S Jul – H Aug); Kale (T) (S Sep – H Nov)
7	Onions (S May – H Jun); Cucumbers (S Jul – H Aug); Spinach (T) (S Oct – H Dec)
8	Beets (S Apr – H Jun); Melons (T) (S Jun – H Sep); Radishes (S Oct – H Nov)

Months: JAN, FEB, MAR, APR, MAY, JUN, JUL, AUG, SEP, OCT, NOV, DEC (each divided into weeks 1, 2, 3, 4)

GROWING ZONE 7

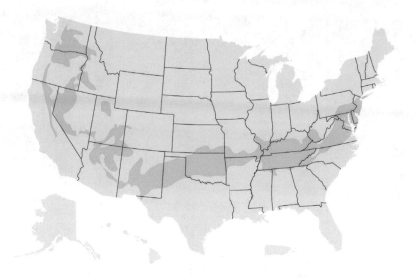

Summary: Growing zone 7 is characterized by having a moderate climate with warm summers and mild winters, allowing for a vast array of gardening opportunities. Annual minimum temperatures in winter months range from 0ºF to 10ºF and annual high temperatures in summer months range from 70ºF to 90ºF. Annual rainfall in growing zone 7 can average 30–50 inches per year, with variations occurring in certain microclimates.

Frost: Zone 7 has quick springs, hot summers, and a relatively short fall season, leading to a long growing season of 180–210 frost-free days. This allows for a quick spring crop planted right around the frost date, a long summer growing season, and a final fall crop planted when the weather is still hot.

- ▸ **Last (spring) frost:** March 31 to April 10
- ▸ **First (fall) frost:** October 20 to November 10

Zone 7 Tips

▸ **Cover your crops with frost cloth in the spring.** Because zone 7 has such a short spring, crops need to be put into the garden early. Frost cloths (with wire hoops for support) can be placed over your crops on cold nights to keep your plants 3–4ºF above the outside temperature and prevent them from freezing.

▸ **Water in the morning.** Summers in zone 7 can be brutally hot. Watering early in the mornings on hot days can reduce the soil temperature throughout the day and prevent crops from bolting (flowering too early due to stressful conditions) or dying.

▸ **Pay attention to pests.** Insects in zone 7 can be intense! Insects attack weak plants, and plants become weak when they don't have enough nutrients in the soil. Treat the soil like a bank account and always deposit when there has been a withdrawal. Add compost at the beginning of every season and organic fertilizers between every planting.

▸ **Retain moisture through mulching.** Mulching a garden bed with straw or wood chips can retain moisture throughout the season. But do not mix the mulch into the soil once the crop is done growing. The mulch will bond with nitrogen in the soil and reduce the soil fertility over time.

Plan Ahead with Your Crop Calendar

Turn the page to see your zone's crop calendar—the master list of when each vegetable should be planted and harvested, according to your frost dates. We've broken the two pages into the spring/summer and the fall seasons to make it easier to read.

ZONE 7	SPRING / SUMMER			
Crop	Indoor Seeding	Outdoor Seeding	Transplanting	Harvest
Arugula		3/1–6/1		4/10–7/1
Basil	3/25–5/1	4/25–8/15	4/25–8/15	6/15–10/15
Beans		4/5–8/15		6/15–10/15
Beets	2/15–4/1	3/15–5/1	3/15–5/1	4/15–6/15
Bok Choy	2/15–4/15	3/15–4/20	3/15–4/15	4/15–6/15
Broccoli	2/15–4/1	3/25–4/25	3/15–5/1	5/15–6/20
Brussels Sprouts	5/1–7/20	5/1–7/20	6/1–8/20	9/1–11/20
Cabbage	2/15–4/1	3/25–4/25	3/15–5/1	5/15–6/20
Carrots		3/7–6/1		5/15–8/15
Cauliflower	2/15–4/1	3/25–4/25	3/15–5/1	5/15–6/20
Chard	2/25–3/25	3/20–4/10	3/25–4/25	4/20–6/25
Chicory	2/15–5/15	3/15–5/15	3/15–6/15	4/15–7/15
Corn		4/25–8/10		7/10–10/25
Cucumbers	3/20–7/15	4/24–7/15	4/21–8/15	6/15–10/15
Eggplant	2/20–7/15	4/20–7/1	4/20–8/15	7/1–10/20
Fennel	2/20–3/30	4/15–5/1	4/1–5/1	4/25–8/1
Garlic				
Green Onions	2/5–3/20	3/15–4/15	3/20–4/30	5/14–6/25
Kale	2/15–3/20	3/25–4/10	3/15–4/20	4/20–6/25
Leeks	1/20–2/15		3/20–4/5	7/15–8/15
Lettuce	2/15–5/5	3/20–5/1	3/15–6/15	4/20–7/15
Melons	4/1–7/1	4/20–7/1	4/20–7/25	7/30–10/10
Mustard		3/1–6/1		4/10–7/1
Okra		4/20–7/20		7/1–10/20
Onions	1/20–2/5	3/1–3/15	3/15–4/15	7/1–9/15
Peppers	2/20–7/15	4/20–7/1	4/20–8/15	7/1–10/20
Peas		3/1–4/15		5/1–7/1
Potatoes		3/15–4/1		6/20–8/1
Radishes		3/1–6/15		4/10–7/20
Spinach	2/5–3/20	3/5–4/20	3/10–4/20	4/5–7/1
Strawberries		3/1–4/15		6/15–8/15
Summer Squash/Zucchini	3/25–7/15	4/21–7/15	4/20–8/7	6/15–10/5
Sweet Potatoes		5/1–6/1		9/20–10/20
Tomatoes	2/20–7/15	4/20–7/1	4/20–8/15	7/1–10/20
Turnips		3/1–6/15		4/20–8/1
Winter Squash/Pumpkins	3/25–7/5	4/25–7/5	4/25–8/1	9/1–10/30

ZONE 7	FALL			
Crop	Indoor Seeding	Outdoor Seeding	Transplanting	Harvest
Arugula		8/15–10/1		9/15–11/15
Basil				
Beans				
Beets	8/1–9/1	8/1–9/1	9/1–10/1	9/20–11/1
Bok Choy	7/20–9/5	8/18–9/15	8/20–10/5	9/20–11/5
Broccoli	7/15–8/1	7/25–8/5	8/15–9/1	9/15–11/15
Brussels Sprouts				
Cabbage	7/15–8/1	7/25–8/5	8/15–9/1	9/15–11/15
Carrots		8/1–9/15		10/1–11/15
Cauliflower	7/15–8/1	7/25–8/5	8/15–9/1	9/15–11/15
Chard	7/25–8/20	8/20–9/1	8/25–9/20	9/20–11/10
Chicory	7/15–8/15	8/15–9/1	8/15–9/15	9/15–11/15
Corn				
Cucumbers				
Eggplant				
Fennel	7/15–8/10	7/25–8/10	8/15–9/10	9/15–10/25
Garlic		10/1–11/20		6/15–7/15
Green Onions	6/25–8/1	6/25–8/1	7/15–9/15	9/1–10/25
Kale	7/20–8/15	8/15–9/1	8/20–9/15	10/1–11/25
Leeks				
Lettuce	7/10–8/20	8/1–9/1	8/10–9/20	9/15–10/25
Melons				
Mustard		8/15–10/1		9/15–11/15
Okra				
Onions				
Peppers				
Peas		8/15–9/1		10/10–11/1
Potatoes				
Radishes		8/10–10/1		9/10–11/15
Spinach	8/10–9/15	9/1–10/15	9/10–10/15	10/1–12/1
Strawberries		9/15–10/30		6/1–7/15
Summer Squash/Zucchini				
Sweet Potatoes				
Tomatoes				
Turnips		8/10–10/1		9/20–11/10
Winter Squash/Pumpkins				

ZONE 7
GARDEN PLAN

To make your first Liberty Garden as simple as possible, we've put together a sample Garden Plan that will guide you every step of the way.

The numbers 1–8 represent the 2' x 2' square plots. You'll plant one vegetable in each. Follow along at the top of the Garden Plan to know what to do each month.

Along the timelines, you'll notice a few key instructions:

S - Ready to Seed
H - Time to Harvest

These instructions are for outdoor seeding only. If you want to seed indoors and transplant (T) to your garden, reference pages 106–107 and adjust your dates accordingly.

Scan the QR code to download a PDF of your sample Garden Plan. You can keep a copy on the fridge or wherever you keep your gardening supplies.

SAMPLE GARDEN PLAN - ZONE 7

S = Seed   H = Harvest   T = Recommended to Seed Indoors and Transplant

1	2	3	4
5	6	7	8

MONTH	JAN	FEB	MAR	APR	MAY	JUN	JUL	AUG	SEP	OCT	NOV	DEC
WEEKS	1 2 3 4	1 2 3 4	1 2 3 4	1 2 3 4	1 2 3 4	1 2 3 4	1 2 3 4	1 2 3 4	1 2 3 4	1 2 3 4	1 2 3 4	1 2 3 4

GARDEN BOXES

Box 1: S Carrots H — S Melons (T) H

Box 2: S Lettuce (T) H — S Summer Squash (T) H — S Carrots H

Box 3: S Radishes H — S Cucumbers — S Beets H

Box 4: S Arugula H — S Tomatoes (T) H — S Arugula H

Box 5: S Broccoli (T) H — S Corn H — S Radishes H

Box 6: S Potatoes — S Basil (T) H — S Lettuce (T) H

Box 7: S Onions — S Beans H — S Spinach (T) H

Box 8: S Beets H — S Peppers (T) H — S Kale (T) H

GROWING ZONE 8

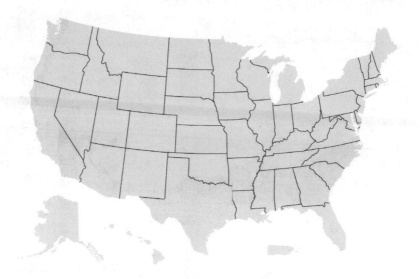

Summary: Growing zone 8 is characterized by a warm climate that has mild winters and hot summers, allowing for a long growing season for gardeners. Annual minimum temperatures in winter months range from 10ºF to 20ºF and annual high temperatures in summer months range from 75ºF to 95ºF. Annual rainfall in growing zone 8 varies depending on geographic location, with less rain falling in dry regions and more rain falling in coastal regions.

Frost: Zone 8 has quick springs, long, hot summers, and short, warm falls, resulting in 225–265 frost-free days. This allows for a wide array of warm season crops to thrive and grow in abundance throughout the year.

- ▸ **Last (spring) frost:** March 12 to March 28
- ▸ **First (fall) frost:** November 7 to November 29

Zone 8 Tips

▸ **Start seeds indoors to protect seedlings from the sun.** Zone 8 has warm summers with intense sun, which can quickly dry out young plants. Starting seeds inside and transplanting them gives you a head start with crops and minimizes the number of days seedlings are exposed to the sun.

▸ **Use shade cloth.** The sun can beat down on tender greens in the garden, especially late in the spring. Use shade cloth to reduce the amount of direct sun on veggies and extend their life in the garden.

▸ **Water in the morning.** Summers in zone 8 can be brutally hot. Watering early in the mornings on hot days can reduce the soil temperature throughout the day and prevent crops from bolting (flowering too early due to stressful conditions) or dying.

▸ **Retain moisture through mulching.** Mulching a garden bed with straw or wood chips can retain moisture throughout the season. But do not mix the mulch into the soil once the crop is done growing. The mulch will bond with nitrogen in the soil and reduce the soil fertility over time.

Plan Ahead with Your Crop Calendar

Turn the page to see your zone's crop calendar—the master list of when each vegetable should be planted and harvested, according to your frost dates. We've broken the two pages into the spring/summer and the fall seasons to make it easier to read.

ZONE 8	SPRING / SUMMER			
Crop	Indoor Seeding	Outdoor Seeding	Transplanting	Harvest
Arugula		2/20–5/15		3/20–6/15
Basil	2/7–5/1	4/1–8/15	4/1–8/21	6/15–11/7
Beans		3/28–8/15		5/20–10/5
Beets	1/20–2/27	2/20–3/15	2/20–3/27	4/15–6/5
Bok Choy	1/25–4/5	2/20–4/1	3/1–5/5	3/30–6/5
Broccoli	1/15–3/1	2/15–3/7	2/25–4/1	3/20–6/10
Brussels Sprouts	1/15–3/15	2/15–3/5	2/25–4/15	4/20–6/25
Cabbage	1/15–3/1	2/15–3/7	2/25–4/1	3/20–6/10
Carrots		2/20–3/20		4/20–6/1
Cauliflower	1/15–3/1	2/15–3/7	2/25–4/1	3/20–6/10
Chard	2/1–3/1	2/20–3/27	3/1–4/1	4/1–5/25
Chicory	1/25–4/5	2/20–4/1	3/1–5/5	3/30–6/5
Corn		4/5–8/20		6/15–11/1
Cucumbers	3/1–8/1	4/1–8/1	4/1–9/1	5/1–10/25
Eggplant	2/1–7/5	4/1–7/5	4/1–8/5	6/20–11/5
Fennel	2/10–3/15	3/20–4/15	3/20–4/25	4/15–7/15
Garlic				
Green Onions	1/15–2/20	2/20–3/15	2/20–3/27	4/15–6/5
Kale	1/20–2/25	3/1–3/15	2/26–4/1	3/20–6/1
Leeks	1/1–2/15	2/20–3/15	3/1–4/1	5/1–7/15
Lettuce	1/25–4/5	2/20–4/1	3/1–5/5	3/30–6/5
Melons	3/1–7/15	4/1–7/15	4/1–8/15	6/15–11/15
Mustard		2/20–5/15		3/20–6/15
Okra		4/1–8/1		7/1–11/1
Onions	1/1–2/15	2/20–3/15	3/1–4/1	5/1–7/15
Peppers	2/1–7/5	4/1–7/5	4/1–8/5	6/20–11/5
Peas		2/15–3/10		4/15–5/25
Potatoes		2/15–3/15		5/15–6/20
Radishes		2/20–5/15		3/20–6/15
Spinach	1/15–3/15	2/20–3/10	2/15–4/15	3/25–6/10
Strawberries				
Summer Squash/Zucchini	3/1–8/1	4/1–8/15	4/1–9/15	5/20–11/1
Sweet Potatoes			4/5–7/15	8/5–11/15
Tomatoes	2/1–7/5	4/1–7/5	4/1–8/5	6/20–11/5
Turnips		2/20–6/1		4/1–7/15
Winter Squash/Pumpkins	3/1–7/30	4/1–7/30	4/1–8/30	6/10–11/5

ZONE 8	FALL			
Crop	Indoor Seeding	Outdoor Seeding	Transplanting	Harvest
Arugula		9/14–10/20		10/14–11/15
Basil				
Beans				
Beets	7/15–9/1	8/19–9/10	8/15–10/1	9/10–11/5
Bok Choy	7/25–9/15	8/25–9/15	8/25–10/15	9/25–11/15
Broccoli	7/25–8/15	8/5–8/20	8/25–9/15	9/25–11/15
Brussels Sprouts	7/25–8/5	7/25–8/5	8/25–9/5	10/30–11/15
Cabbage	7/25–8/15	8/5–8/20	8/25–9/15	9/25–11/15
Carrots		8/15–9/15		10/15–12/1
Cauliflower	7/25–8/15	8/5–8/20	8/25–9/15	9/25–11/15
Chard				
Chicory	7/25–9/15	8/25–9/15	8/25–10/15	9/25–11/15
Corn				
Cucumbers				
Eggplant				
Fennel	7/10–8/15	8/5–8/25	8/10–9/15	9/15–11/15
Garlic		11/15–12/10		6/1–7/20
Green Onions	7/10–9/1	8/19–9/10	8/15–10/1	9/10–11/5
Kale	8/1–9/15	8/25–9/15	9/1–10/15	10/1–12/1
Leeks				
Lettuce	7/25–9/15	8/25–9/15	8/25–10/15	9/25–11/15
Melons				
Mustard		9/14–10/20		10/14–11/15
Okra				
Onions				
Peppers				
Peas		8/25–9/15		10/25–11/25
Potatoes				
Radishes		9/14–10/20		10/14–11/15
Spinach	8/15–9/20	9/1–10/15	9/10–10/20	10/1–12/1
Strawberries			9/1–11/1	6/1–8/1
Summer Squash/Zucchini				
Sweet Potatoes				
Tomatoes				
Turnips		9/14–10/15		10/14–11/25
Winter Squash/Pumpkins				

ZONE 8
GARDEN PLAN

To make your first Liberty Garden as simple as possible, we've put together a sample Garden Plan that will guide you every step of the way.

The numbers 1–8 represent the 2' x 2' square plots. You'll plant one vegetable in each. Follow along at the top of the Garden Plan to know what to do each month.

Along the timelines, you'll notice a few key instructions:

S - Ready to Seed

H - Time to Harvest

These instructions are for outdoor seeding only. If you want to seed indoors and transplant (T) to your garden, reference pages 106–107 and adjust your dates accordingly.

Scan the QR code to download a PDF of your sample Garden Plan. You can keep a copy on the fridge or wherever you keep your gardening supplies.

SAMPLE GARDEN PLAN - ZONE 8

S = Seed   H = Harvest   T = Recommended to Seed Indoors and Transplant

GARDEN BOXES	MONTH	JAN				FEB				MAR				APR				MAY				JUN				JUL				AUG				SEP				OCT				NOV				DEC			
	WEEKS	1	2	3	4	1	2	3	4	1	2	3	4	1	2	3	4	1	2	3	4	1	2	3	4	1	2	3	4	1	2	3	4	1	2	3	4	1	2	3	4	1	2	3	4	1	2	3	4
	1	Carrots · Melons (T) · Kale (T)																																															
	2	Lettuce (T) · Radishes · Summer Squash (T) · Beans · Radishes																																															
	3	Radishes · Cucumbers · Basil (T) · Spinach (T)																																															
	4	Arugula · Tomatoes (T) · Peas																																															
	5	Broccoli (T) · Potatoes · Corn · Carrots																																															
	6	Onions · Cucumbers · Lettuce (T)																																															
	7	Beets · Peppers (T) · Tomatoes (T)																																															
	8	Beets · Broccoli (T)																																															

GROWING ZONE 9

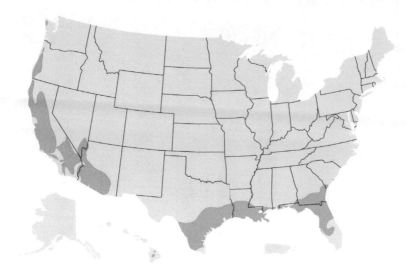

Summary: Growing zone 9 is characterized by mild, warm winters and long, hot summers. Being one of the warmest zones in the country, zone 9 experiences annual minimum temperatures around 20ºF to 30ºF in winter months and annual high temperatures around 80ºF to 95ºF. Annual rainfall in zone 9 is hard to predict, given the vast geographical range that zone 9 covers—from California and southern Arizona to Florida and southern Louisiana.

Frost: Zone 9 has a very short winter and long, hot summers, resulting in 270–300 frost-free days. This gives you the opportunity to grow a vast number of vegetables virtually all year long.

- ▸ **Last (spring) frost:** February 6 to February 28
- ▸ **First (fall) frost:** November 25 to December 15

Zone 9 Tips

- **Use shade cloth.** Growing vegetables in zone 9 can be very challenging with the amount of sun exposure that the vegetables endure. Shade cloths can reduce the amount of UV light that the plants are receiving and lower the temperature under the cloth. This can help plants like broccoli, cabbage, and greens thrive during summer.

- **Water early in the morning.** In growing zone 9, the high temperatures can make plants bolt—meaning they go to seed prematurely due to stressful conditions. Reducing the soil temperature, which allows the roots to stay cool, can significantly increase the success rate of the vegetable. On the hottest days, water deeply early in the mornings before the sun comes up to help tender plants cope with the heat.

- **Avoid the heat.** Treat spring and fall as your main growing seasons. You can plant a few crops like tomatoes, peppers, and melons that can handle the heat during the height of the summer, but don't plant greens during the summer unless you feel up for the challenge.

- **Plant vegetables that thrive in your area.** Choose varieties of vegetables that are suited for hotter climates. When planning and buying seeds, look for key phrases like "bolt resistant" or "adapted to hot climates."

Plan Ahead with Your Crop Calendar

Turn the page to see your zone's crop calendar—the master list of when each vegetable should be planted and harvested, according to your frost dates. We've broken the two pages into the spring/summer and the fall seasons to make it easier to read.

ZONE 9	SPRING / SUMMER			
Crop	Indoor Seeding	Outdoor Seeding	Transplanting	Harvest
Arugula		2/1–5/1		3/1–6/1
Basil	2/10–9/1	3/15–9/1	3/15–10/1	4/20–11/25
Beans		3/20–9/20		5/20–11/25
Beets	1/15–3/1	2/15–3/10	2/15–4/1	3/15–5/10
Bok Choy	1/15–3/15	2/10–3/1	2/15–4/15	3/15–5/20
Broccoli	1/5–2/20	2/10–2/25	2/15–3/20	3/15–5/20
Brussels Sprouts	1/15–2/15	2/1–2/20	2/15–3/15	5/20–6/30
Cabbage	1/5–2/20	2/10–2/25	2/15–3/20	3/15–5/20
Carrots		2/1–3/5		4/1–5/15
Cauliflower	1/5–2/20	2/10–2/25	2/15–3/20	3/15–5/20
Chard	1/20–2/15	2/10–2/25	2/20–3/15	3/20–5/1
Chicory	1/15–3/15	2/10–3/1	2/15–4/15	3/15–5/20
Corn		3/15–9/1		6/5–11/15
Cucumbers	2/15–8/15	3/15–9/1	3/15–9/15	5/15–11/25
Eggplant	1/15–7/15	3/15–7/15	3/15–9/15	5/15–11/25
Fennel	1/20–3/1	3/1–4/1	2/20–4/1	3/25–7/1
Garlic				
Green Onions				
Kale	1/5–2/20	2/5–2/25	2/5–3/20	3/7–5/5
Leeks	12/25–2/1	2/10–3/1	2/10–3/15	4/25–6/1
Lettuce	1/15–3/15	2/10–3/1	2/15–4/15	3/15–5/20
Melons	2/15–8/10	3/15–8/5	3/15–9/5	5/20–11/20
Mustard		2/1–5/1		3/1–6/1
Okra		3/15–7/15		6/20–11/15
Onions	12/25–2/1	2/10–3/1	2/10–3/15	4/25–6/1
Peppers	1/15–7/15	3/15–7/15	3/15–9/15	5/15–11/25
Peas		2/1–3/1		5/1–6/1
Potatoes		2/1–3/5		5/1–6/15
Radishes		2/1–5/1		3/1–6/1
Spinach	1/15–3/1	2/20–3/15	2/15–4/1	3/15–5/15
Strawberries				
Summer Squash/Zucchini	2/15–9/1	3/15–9/1	3/15–10/1	5/10–11/25
Sweet Potatoes			3/15–8/15	6/20–12/1
Tomatoes	1/15–7/15	3/15–7/15	3/15–9/15	5/15–11/25
Turnips		2/1–5/1		3/15–6/15
Winter Squash/Pumpkins	2/15–8/20	3/15–8/20	3/15–8/20	5/20–11/25

ZONE 9	FALL			
Crop	Indoor Seeding	Outdoor Seeding	Transplanting	Harvest
Arugula		9/20–11/20		10/20–1/1
Basil				
Beans				
Beets	8/20–9/10	8/25–10/1	8/20–10/10	10/20–12/1
Bok Choy	8/5–9/20	9/5–10/5	9/5–10/20	10/5–12/1
Broccoli	8/1–9/8	8/10–9/5	9/1–10/8	10/1–12/5
Brussels Sprouts	7/15–8/15	7/25–8/15	8/15–9/15	10/25–12/15
Cabbage	8/1–9/8	8/10–9/5	9/1–10/8	10/1–12/5
Carrots		8/25–9/20		10/25–12/1
Cauliflower	8/1–9/8	8/10–9/5	9/1–10/8	10/1–12/5
Chard	8/15–9/8	9/1–10/1	9/15–10/8	10/15–12/5
Chicory	8/5–9/20	9/5–10/5	9/5–10/20	10/5–11/25
Corn				
Cucumbers				
Eggplant				
Fennel	7/20–9/15	8/15–9/15	8/20–10/15	9/25–12/1
Garlic		11/25–1/1		6/1–7/20
Green Onions				
Kale	8/10–9/15	9/5–10/1	9/10–10/15	10/10–12/30
Leeks				
Lettuce	8/5–9/20	9/5–10/5	9/5–10/20	10/5–11/25
Melons				
Mustard		9/20–11/20		10/20–1/1
Okra				
Onions				
Peppers				
Peas		9/1–10/5		10/25–12/5
Potatoes				
Radishes		9/20–11/20		10/20–1/1
Spinach	8/15–9/20	9/1–10/15	9/10–11/1	10/1–12/20
Strawberries			9/20–11/15	6/1–8/1
Summer Squash/Zucchini				
Sweet Potatoes				
Tomatoes				
Turnips		9/20–11/20		10/25–1/1
Winter Squash/Pumpkins				

ZONE 9
GARDEN PLAN

To make your first Liberty Garden as simple as possible, we've put together a sample Garden Plan that will guide you every step of the way.

The numbers 1—8 represent the 2' x 2' square plots. You'll plant one vegetable in each. Follow along at the top of the Garden Plan to know what to do each month.

Along the timelines, you'll notice a few key instructions:

S - Ready to Seed

H - Time to Harvest

These instructions are for outdoor seeding only. If you want to seed indoors and transplant (T) to your garden, reference pages 106—107 and adjust your dates accordingly.

Scan the QR code to download a PDF of your sample Garden Plan. You can keep a copy on the fridge or wherever you keep your gardening supplies.

S = Seed   H = Harvest   T = Recommended to Seed Indoors and Transplant

1	2	3	4
5	6	7	8

GARDEN BOXES

Box	Plantings (S = Seed, H = Harvest)
1	Carrots (S Feb – H May); Melons (T) (S May – H Aug); Kale (T) (S Sep – H Dec)
2	Lettuce (T) (S Feb – H Mar); Summer Squash (T) (S Apr – H Jun); Beans (S Jun – H Aug); Beets (S Sep – H Nov)
3	Radishes (S Feb – H Mar); Cucumbers (S Apr – H Jun); Basil (T) (S Jun – H Aug); Peas (S Sep – H Nov)
4	Arugula (S Feb – H Mar); Tomatoes (T) (S Apr – H Jul); Carrots (S Sep – H Nov)
5	Broccoli (T) (S Feb – H Apr); Corn (S May – H Jul); Beans (S Jul – H Sep); Radishes (S Oct – H Nov)
6	Potatoes (S Feb – H May); Cucumbers (S Jun – H Aug); Spinach (T) (S Oct – H Nov)
7	Onions (S Feb – H May); Tomatoes (T) (S Jun – H Oct); Lettuce (T) (S Nov)
8	Peas (S Feb – H Apr); Peppers (T) (S Apr – H Aug); Broccoli (T) (S Sep – H Nov)

Months: JAN, FEB, MAR, APR, MAY, JUN, JUL, AUG, SEP, OCT, NOV, DEC (Weeks 1–4 each)

SPACING GUIDE

As you plant, follow the instructions below for proper spacing and placement. At first, you'll overplant some crops for each 2' x 2' square—since not every plant will make it. Once your seeds have germinated (broken through the surface and sprouted), refer to each plant's spacing guide and thin your seedlings, plucking out the necessary number to give the remaining plants plenty of space (some plants, like arugula, mustard, and radishes, likely won't need to be thinned).

Arugula

- ▸ Plant arugula in five rows with 48 seeds per row.
- ▸ Each square should produce 240 plants.
- ▸ Your estimated harvest per square is 2 pounds.

Basil

- ▸ Plant basil in five rows with six seeds per row.
- ▸ If you're transplanting basil to your garden, place each plant 12 inches apart (four plants can fit in each square).
- ▸ You can expect to grow four basil plants per square.
- ▸ Your estimated harvest per square is 2 pounds.

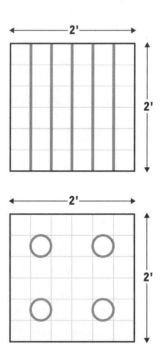

Beans

▸ Plant beans in two rows with 12 seeds per row.

▸ If you're transplanting beans to your garden, place each plant 5 inches apart.

▸ Each square should produce eight plants.

▸ Your estimated harvest per square is 2.5 pounds.

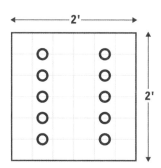

Beets

▸ Plant beets in two rows with 12 seeds per row.

▸ If you're transplanting beets to your garden, place each plant 5 inches apart.

▸ Each square should produce eight plants.

▸ Your estimated harvest per square is eight large beet heads.

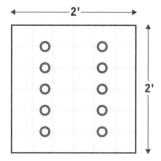

Bok Choy

▸ Plant bok choy in three rows with six seeds per row.

▸ If you're transplanting bok choy to your garden, place each plant 6 inches apart.

▸ Each square should produce nine plants.

▸ Your estimated harvest is nine heads.

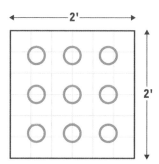

Broccoli

- Plant broccoli in one row with three seeds (or transplant one plant per square).
- Each square should produce one plant.
- Your estimated harvest per square is one large head.

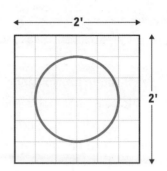

Brussels Sprouts

- Plant Brussels sprouts in one row with three seeds (or transplant one plant per square).
- Each square should produce one plant.
- Your estimated harvest per square is one large stalk.

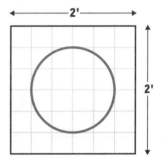

Cabbage

- Plant cabbage in one row with three seeds (or transplant one plant per square).
- Each square should produce one plant.
- Your estimated harvest per square is one large head.

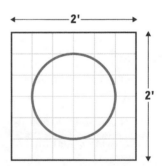

Carrots

▸ Plant carrots in three rows with 16 seeds per row.

▸ Each square should produce 48 plants.

▸ Your estimated harvest per square is 2 pounds.

Cauliflower

▸ Plant cauliflower in one row with three seeds (or transplant one plant per square).

▸ Each square should produce one plant.

▸ Your estimated harvest per square is one large head.

Chard

▸ Plant chard in two rows with three seeds per row.

▸ If you're transplanting chard to your garden, place each plant 12 inches apart.

▸ Each square should produce four plants.

▸ Your estimated harvest per square is 2–3 pounds.

Chicory/Radicchio

- Plant chicory or radicchio in two rows with three seeds per row.
- If you're transplanting chicory or radicchio to your garden, place each plant 12 inches apart.
- Each square should produce four plants.
- Your estimated harvest per square is four large heads.

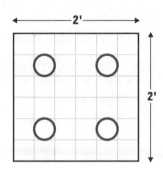

Corn

- Plant corn in one row with three seeds.
- If you're transplanting corn to your garden, place each plant 12 inches apart.
- Each square should produce one or two plants.
- Your estimated harvest per square is one to four ears.

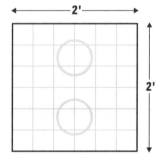

Cucumbers

- Plant cucumber in one row with three seeds (or transplant one plant per square).
- Each square should produce one plant.
- Your estimated harvest per square is 8–12 cucumbers.
- For best results, set up a trellis for your cucumbers to grow on.

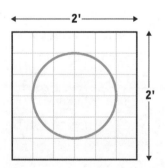

Eggplant

▸ Plant eggplant in one row with three seeds (or transplant one plant per square).

▸ Each square should produce one plant.

▸ Your estimated harvest per square is four to six eggplants.

▸ For best results, set up a trellis for your eggplant to grow on.

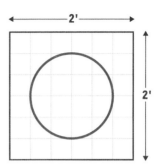

Fennel

▸ Plant fennel in three rows with six seeds per row.

▸ If you're transplanting fennel to your garden, place each plant 6 inches apart.

▸ Each square should produce nine plants.

▸ Your estimated harvest per square is nine bulbs.

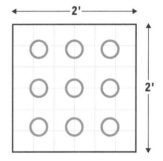

Garlic

▸ Plant garlic in three rows with four seeds per row.

▸ If you're transplanting garlic to your garden, place each plant 6 inches apart.

▸ Each square should produce nine plants.

▸ Your estimated harvest per square is nine bulbs.

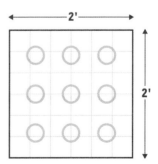

Green Onions

▸ Plant green onions in three rows with 48 seeds per row.

▸ Each square should produce 144 plants.

▸ Your estimated harvest per square is 3 pounds.

Kale

▸ Plant kale in two rows with four seeds per row.

▸ If you're transplanting kale to your garden, place each plant 12 inches apart.

▸ Each square should produce four plants.

▸ Your estimated harvest per square is 2–3 pounds.

Leeks

▸ Plant leeks in three rows with nine seeds per row.

▸ If you're transplanting leeks to your garden, place each plant 6 inches apart.

▸ Each square should produce nine plants.

▸ Your estimated harvest per square is nine large heads.

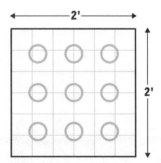

Lettuce

- ▸ Plant lettuce in two rows with six seeds per row.
- ▸ If you're transplanting lettuce to your garden, place each plant 10 inches apart.
- ▸ Each square should produce four to five plants.
- ▸ Your estimated harvest per square is four to five large heads.

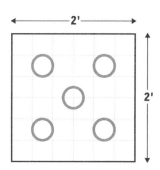

Melons

- ▸ Plant one melon seed in each square (or transplant one if seeding indoors).
- ▸ Your melon plant will likely outgrow the 2' x 2' square, which is okay. For best results, set up a trellis for your melon to grow on, or allow it to expand outside the bed.
- ▸ Your estimated harvest is two to three melons per plant.

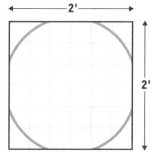

Mustard

- Plant mustard in five rows with 48 seeds per row.
- If you're transplanting mustard to your garden, place each plant a half-inch apart.
- Each square should produce 240 plants.
- Your estimated harvest per square is 2 pounds.

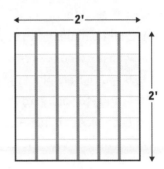

Okra

- Plant okra in one row with three seeds (or transplant one plant per square).
- Each square should produce one plant.
- Your estimated harvest is 20–25 okra pods.

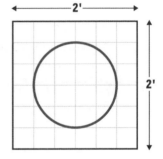

Onions

- Plant onions in two rows with 12 seeds per row.
- If you're transplanting onions to your garden, place each plant 6 inches apart.
- Each square should produce eight plants.
- Your estimated harvest is eight large onions.

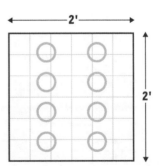

Peppers

- ▸ Plant peppers in one row with three seeds (or transplant one plant per square).
- ▸ Each square should produce one plant.
- ▸ Your estimated harvest is 7–10 large peppers or 20–49 small peppers.
- ▸ For best results, set up a trellis for your peppers to grow on.

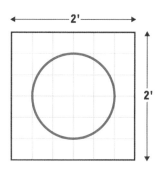

Peas

- ▸ Plant peas in one row with 12 seeds.
- ▸ If you're transplanting peas to your garden, place each plant 3 inches apart.
- ▸ Each square should produce six plants.
- ▸ Your estimated harvest is 1.25 pounds.
- ▸ For best results, set up a trellis for your peas to grow on.

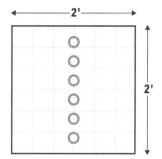

Potatoes

- ▸ Plant potatoes in one row with two seeds.
- ▸ If you're transplanting potatoes to your garden, place each plant 8 inches apart.
- ▸ Each square should produce two plants.
- ▸ Your estimated harvest is 4–5 pounds.
- ▸ For every 8 inches that your potato plant grows, pile up soil or mulch around its base (a process known as *hilling*). Covering the tubers (the part of the potato plant we eat) will stimulate growth and protect them from direct exposure to the sun.

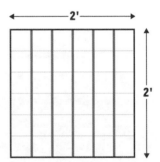

Radishes

- ▸ Plant radishes in five rows with 32 seeds per row.
- ▸ If you're transplanting radishes to your garden, place each plant 1 inch apart.
- ▸ Each square should produce 110 plants.
- ▸ Your estimated harvest per square is 100 radishes.

Spinach

- ▸ Plant spinach in four rows with 22 seeds per row.
- ▸ If you're transplanting spinach to your garden, place each plant 3 inches apart.
- ▸ Each square should produce 21 plants.
- ▸ Your estimated harvest per square is 2–3 pounds.

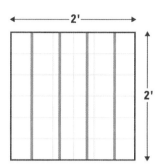

Strawberries

- ▸ Plant strawberries in two rows with two seeds per row.
- ▸ If you're transplanting strawberries to your garden, place each plant 12 inches apart.
- ▸ Each square should produce four plants.
- ▸ Your estimated harvest per square is 2–3 pounds.

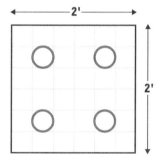

Summer Squash/Zucchini

- ▸ Plant summer squash or zucchini in one row with three seeds (or transplant one plant per square).
- ▸ Each square should produce one plant.
- ▸ Your estimated harvest is 6–10 squash.

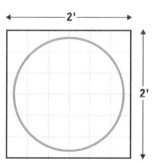

Sweet Potatoes

▸ Plant one sweet potato slip per square (or transplant one plant per square).

▸ Each square should produce one plant.

▸ Your estimated harvest is 2–3 pounds.

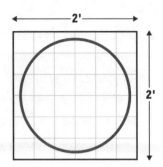

Tomatoes

▸ Plant tomatoes in one row with two seeds (or transplant one plant per square if seeding indoor or starting from a plant).

▸ Each square should produce one plant.

▸ Your estimated harvest is 20 large tomatoes or 150 cherry tomatoes.

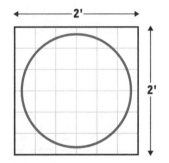

Turnips

▸ Plant turnips in four rows with 24 seeds per row.

▸ If you're transplanting turnips to your garden, place each plant 1.5 inches apart.

▸ Each square should produce 64 plants.

▸ Your estimated harvest is 64 turnips.

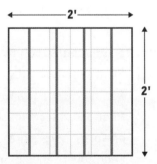

Winter Squash/Pumpkins

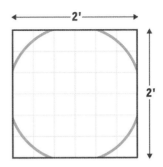

- ▸ Plant one winter squash or pumpkin in each square (or transplant one plant per square).
- ▸ Your winter squash or pumpkin will likely outgrow the 2' x 2' square, which is okay. For best results, set up a trellis for it to grow on, or allow it to expand outside the bed.
- ▸ Your estimated harvest is 2–5 squash per plant.
- ▸ For best results, allow your winter squash or pumpkins to grow outside of the bed.

INDOOR SEEDING

Starting seeds indoors may sound like an added burden to gardening, but it will make growing much easier in the long run! It results in a much higher rate of germination, ensuring that only strong, healthy plants go into the garden and minimizing the amount of loss in the first 30 days of a plant's life.

Indoor seeding is also key to getting more out of your garden in a single season! While the plants in the garden are finishing their growing cycle and getting ready to be harvested, the next plant going into the garden can already be 30 days old, giving you a month's head start on the next crop.

To learn how to start seeds indoors and transplant them to your garden, scan the QR code and watch the videos on our tutorial page. You'll find other resources on seeds there, too!

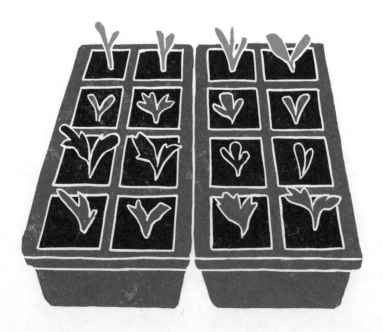

Transplant List

These plants thrive when started indoors and transplanted into your garden.

Crop	Number of Days Before Transplant Date to Start Seeds Indoors
Basil	30
Beets	30–40
Bok Choy	30
Broccoli	30–40
Brussels Sprouts	30–40
Cabbage	30–40
Cauliflower	30–40
Chard	30
Chicory	30
Cucumbers	21–28
Eggplant	30–60
Fennel	30
Green Onions	45
Kale	30
Leeks	50–75
Lettuce	30
Melons	21–28
Okra	30–40
Onions	50–75
Peppers	30–60
Spinach	30
Summer Squash/Zucchini	21–28
Tomatoes	30–60
Winter Squash/Pumpkins	21–28

Gratitude

This book would not have been possible without the support and encouragement of many people. First and foremost, I want to honor my beautiful wife, Amy: You are my better 9/10ths and my partner in everything I do. You are my forever companion, walking with me through endless ideas, adventures, and opportunities. I also want to thank our children: Gabriel, who has inspired me to be a lifelong learner, and Ava, who helps me find joy in everyday life. You three have given me decades of tireless love, encouragement, and wisdom. Your support in the pursuit of this grand dream is yet another example of that goodness and grace. You are my heroes and my greatest blessing.

While inspiration for Liberty Gardens Project came from many sources, my wife and I would like to thank a few folks in particular: Gabe and Rebekah Lyons of THINQ, Joey Lankford of Cul2vate, and Ryan and Gerda Audagnotti of Acres of Love. Thank you for helping us grow Liberty Gardens Project from an idea to a reality.

As an amateur gardener, I'm highly aware of the role the past plays in my present, and I'm humbled to be a part of the larger growing community. I owe a lot to the subject matter experts in the gardening space who have gone before us, rolled up their sleeves, and documented their journey. Without their pioneering work, I'm confident that *Liberty Gardens Guidebook*—and hundreds more like it—may never have been written. Those who have heeded the call to encourage, train, and mentor others are owed significant gratitude. Thank you to everyone who has taught me in person and online.

I would like to acknowledge the Liberty Gardens Project team members, specifically Peyton Cypress, Leila Giannetti, Miriam Wilson, Garrett Abbott, and Mary Wright. Thank you for making this guidebook possible and continuing to assist in the movement we are creating. We would also like to call out those who have contributed significant efforts and excellence to the launch of the guidebook, website, social media, and organization. Thank you to Rachel Miller, Weylon Smith, Kelsey Chapman, April Cox, Erik Olsen, James Brown, and Jordan Russ. Your ability to rise to this moment and provide sharp insights made this book a much better version of itself.

And finally, I would like to thank the Almighty Lord—the one who made the very first garden. This world is your masterpiece, and I marvel at the mystery of your design. The earth's capacity for regenerative creativity reflects the wonders of science and the depth of your love. At Liberty Gardens Project, we desire to steward the gift you've entrusted to us as you intended. Everything listed above, and more, is because of your grace and mercy in my life.

Cheers!

Randal Clark
Liberty Gardens Project

"Everyone will sit under their own vine and under their own fig tree, and no one will make them afraid…"
Micah 4:4 (NIV)

"Build houses and settle down; plant gardens and eat what they produce."
Jeremiah 29:5 (NIV)

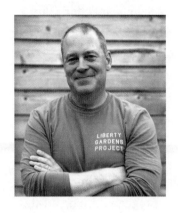

ABOUT THE AUTHOR

Randal Clark is a passionate advocate for community reliance, healthy living, and the transformative power of gardening. After founding, running, and successfully selling several businesses, Randal turned his attention to creating a private family farm in Middle Tennessee. This farm, built on holistic, regenerative, and uncompromising methods, gave him a deep understanding of the critical food challenges we all face today.

Recognizing that many people feel overwhelmed by the idea of growing their own food, Randal applied his expertise and research into developing a beginner-friendly solution. The Liberty Gardens Project was born, providing simple, actionable steps for anyone—regardless of space or experience—to start growing their own produce. His passion project culminated in the *Liberty Gardens Guidebook*, a resource designed to inspire and empower people to create "Gardens everywhere."

Randal enjoys life on the farm with his wife, Amy, and their family, where they harvest fresh, homegrown food from their farm and share it with their community. His mission is simple yet profound: to help everyone discover the joy, freedom, and health that come with growing something, no matter where they are.

"Grow something. Grow anything. Gardens everywhere."

WE WANT TO CELEBRATE YOUR WORK!

Liberty Gardens Project is your #1 fan. Scan this QR code regularly for surprise offers—and keep up the good work!

Cheers!